ACCESS YOUR ONLINE RESOURCES

Navigating Eating, Drinking and Swallowing in Adults is accompanied by a number of printable online materials, designed to ensure that this resource best supports your professional needs.

Go to https://resourcecentre.routledge.com/speechmark and click on the cover of this book.

Answer the question prompt using your copy of the book to gain access to the online content.

NAVIGATING EATING, DRINKING AND SWALLOWING IN ADULTS

This book offers accessible and concise information to enable both student and qualified clinicians to navigate essential eating, drinking and swallowing (EDS) knowledge and equip them to meet relevant clinical competencies.

Arranged alphabetically, the book provides an A to Z of EDS assessment and management in adults, guiding readers through key aspects, from aetiologies to xerostomia and from cranial nerve assessments to videofluoroscopy. This dip in, dip out resource is packed with information of immediate clinical relevance, facilitating synthesis between theory and practice, and encourages readers to view their clients in a holistic, person-centred way. It contains printable resources and concludes with a useful appendix providing worked examples of clinical scenarios.

Divided into 50 tips to enhance practice, this pocket-sized guide is an essential resource for all trainee and newly qualified speech and language therapists, as well as more experienced clinicians moving into the field.

Sophie MacKenzie has practised as a speech and language therapist (SLT) in both acute and rehabilitation settings. She began her first academic role in 2007, combining clinical management of the acute SLT team at Maidstone and Tunbridge Wells NHS Trust with teaching at the University of Greenwich and Canterbury Christ Church University. She moved into full-time academia in 2010 and has taught EDS to both undergraduate and postgraduate pre-registration students, as well as post-registration master's students, at City St Georges, University of London. Her PhD focused on exploring spirituality with people with expressive aphasia, and person-centred and holistic care remains her passion, as well as the nurturing of future clinicians. Sophie is the author of *Working with Adults with Eating, Drinking and Swallowing Needs* and is currently a senior lecturer in SLT at Health Sciences University, UK.

NAVIGATING SPEECH AND LANGUAGE THERAPY

Navigating the field of speech and language therapy can seem overwhelming to students and newly qualified therapists. This series is designed to provide concise, entry-level summaries of key areas in speech and language therapy, providing basic insight into a specific area of therapy. Comprising practical advice and guidance from experts in the field, the books cover topics such as assessment, therapy, psychological approaches and onward referral. These are useful tools for anyone new to speech and language therapy or building confidence in their field.

Navigating Eating, Drinking and Swallowing in Adults
50 Top Tips from A-Z
Sophie MacKenzie

Navigating Aphasia
100 Useful Points for Speech and Language Therapists
Tessa Ackerman

Navigating Speech Sound Disorders in Children
50 Essential Strategies and Resources
Kathryn Murrell

Navigating Trans Voicing
50 Tips, Techniques and Fundamentals for Speech and Language Therapists
Matthew Mills and Natasha Stavropoulos

Navigating Voice Disorders
Around the Larynx in 50 Tips
Carolyn Andrews

NAVIGATING EATING, DRINKING AND SWALLOWING IN ADULTS

50 TOP TIPS FROM A-Z

Sophie MacKenzie

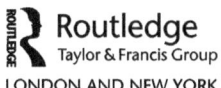

Routledge
Taylor & Francis Group
LONDON AND NEW YORK

Designed cover image: Getty Images

First published 2026
by Routledge
4 Park Square, Milton Park, Abingdon, Oxon OX14 4RN

and by Routledge
605 Third Avenue, New York, NY 10158

Routledge is an imprint of the Taylor & Francis Group, an informa business

© 2026 Sophie MacKenzie

The right of Sophie MacKenzie to be identified as author of this work has been asserted in accordance with sections 77 and 78 of the Copyright, Designs and Patents Act 1988.

All rights reserved. The purchase of this copyright material confers the right on the purchasing institution to photocopy or download pages which bear the support material icon and a copyright line at the bottom of the page. No other parts of this book may be reprinted or reproduced or utilised in any form or by any electronic, mechanical, or other means, now known or hereafter invented, including photocopying and recording, or in any information storage or retrieval system, without permission in writing from the publishers.

Trademark notice: Product or corporate names may be trademarks or registered trademarks, and are used only for identification and explanation without intent to infringe.

British Library Cataloguing-in-Publication Data
A catalogue record for this book is available from the British Library

ISBN: 978-1-032-77017-8 (hbk)
ISBN: 978-1-032-77015-4 (pbk)
ISBN: 978-1-003-48087-7 (ebk)

DOI: 10.4324/9781003480877

Typeset in Times New Roman
by Apex CoVantage, LLC

Access the Support Material: https://resourcecentre.routledge.com/speechmark

For my beautiful sisters, Alexandra and Rachel

CONTENTS

List of abbreviations	xv
Acknowledgements	xviii
Introduction	xix

A — 1

Aetiologies	1
Neurogenic	1
Structural	2
Functional	7
Ageing	8
Learning disability and physical disability	8
Anatomy and physiology	8
Key structures	9
Musculature	11
Physiology	12
Oral preparatory stage	12
Oral stage	13
Pharyngeal stage	14
Oesophageal stage	15
Aspiration, laryngeal penetration and choking	15
Aspiration pneumonia	17

B — 18

Bolus	18
Buccinator, buccal tension	19

C — 21

Cervical auscultation	21
Clinical history	22

Clinical reasoning	22
Judith	25
Prakash	26
Oral hygiene exam	28
CNA	29
Laryngeal palpation	29
Oral trials	29
Tommy	30
Dervla	30
Clinical swallow examination (CSE)	31
Compensatory strategies	32
Head/body positioning	32
Swallow manoeuvres	34
Changes to the environment	35
Helping the person to eat and drink	35
Utensils	36
Texture modification	37
Cranial nerves, cranial nerve assessment (CNA)	37

D   46

Dentition	46
Direct therapy techniques	47
Dysphagia	47

E   54

End-of-life	54
Enteral feeding	55
Epiglottis/epiglottic retroversion	57

F   60

Fibreoptic endoscopic evaluation of swallowing (FEES)	60

G   63

Goal-setting and measuring outcomes	63

H — 68

Holistic EDS practice — 68
  Psychological aspects — 69
  Social aspects — 71
  Spiritual/religious aspects — 71
  Cultural aspects — 73
  Supporting clients' psychological, social,
    spiritual/religious and cultural needs — 74
  Mitigating the power differential — 74
  Narrative in EDS needs — 75
  chaos — 76
  restitution — 76
  quest — 77

I — 79

International Classification of Disability,
  Functioning and Health (ICF) — 79
International Dysphagia Diet Standardisation
  Initiative (IDDSI) — 80

J — 83

Joint working — 83
  Carer — 84
  Chaplain — 84
  Client — 85
  Dietitian — 85
  Doctor — 85
  Healthcare assistant — 86
  Nurse — 86
  Occupational therapist — 87
  Pharmacist — 87
  Physiotherapist — 88
  Physiotherapist (respiratory) — 88
  Psychologist — 89

Radiologist	89
Radiographer	89
Speech and language therapy assistant	90
Speech and language therapy student	90

K 92

Keep reflecting and learning	92
Reflection	92
Continuing professional development (CPD)	92
Killian's triangle	94

L 95

Larynx	95
Laryngeal anatomy, physiology, function and innervation	95
Laryngeal or hyolaryngeal excursion	97
Laryngeal palpation	97
Hyolaryngeal excursion and treatment options	99
Cough and cough testing	100

M 103

Mastication	103
Medication	103

N 105

Nil by mouth (NBM)/*nil per os* (NPO)	105
Neurological underpinnings	105

O 109

Odynophagia	109
Oral hygiene, oral examination and oral care	109

P 112

Positioning	112
Presbyphagia	114

Osteophytes	114
Pulse oximetry	116

Q — 118

Questions to ask the client and carer (case history)	118

R — 122

Residue	122
Oral residue	122
Pharyngeal residue	123
Risk	124

S — 126

Session planning	126

T — 129

Tastes for pleasure	129
Three tenets of EDS management	129
Tracheostomy	130
Decannulation	133
EDS assessment	134
EDS management	136
Key EDS differences between tracheostomy and laryngectomy	137

U — 138

Uvula	138

V — 140

Videofluoroscopy (VF)	140
What is it?	140
What happens during the procedure?	140
Why might you refer a client?	143
Pros and cons	144
Personnel	145

Consent	145
Safety considerations	146
Writing the report	147

W · 148

Water – protocols and tests	148
Frazier Free Water Protocol	148
Timed Water Swallow Test (TWST)	149

X · 151

Xerostomia, sialorrhoea and salivation	151
Xerostomia	152
Sialorrhoea	153

Y · 155

Yoghurt	155
Your supervision and support	155

Z · 157

Zoom or EDS assessment and management via telehealth	157

Appendix	**160**
References	**175**
Index	**181**

LIST OF ABBREVIATIONS

ADL	Activities of daily living
AP	Anterior-posterior
Ax	Assessment
CA	Cervical auscultation
CN	Cranial nerve
CNA	Cranial nerve assessment
CPD	Continuing professional development
CSE	Clinical swallow examination
CT	Computed tomography
DH	Drug history
DOB	Date of birth
EDAR	Eating and drinking with acknowledged risk
EDS	Eating, drinking and swallowing
EEG	Electroencephalogram
EMST	Expiratory muscle strength training
ENT	Ear, nose, and throat
EoL	End of life
FEES	Fibreoptic endoscopic evaluation of swallowing
FOIS	Functional Oral Intake Scale
GCS	Glasgow Coma Scale
GP	General practitioner
HCA	Healthcare assistant
HCPC	Health and Care Professions Council
HME	Heat moisture exchanger
HPC	History of the presenting condition
HR	Heart rate
ICF	International Classification of Disability, Functioning and Health

IDDSI		International Dysphagia Diet Standardisation Initiative
IV		Intravenous
L		Left
LDoL		Last days of life
LMN		Lower motor neurone
LSVT®		Lee Silverman Voice Treatment
MDT		Multidisciplinary team
MEBDT		Modified Evans Blue Dye Test
MND		Motor neurone disease
MRI		Magnetic resonance imaging
Mx		Management
NBM		Nil by mouth
NGT		Nasogastric tube
NIDDM		Non-insulin-dependent diabetes mellitus
NPO		*Nil per os*
NQP		Newly qualified practitioner
O/E		On examination
OT		Occupational therapist
OTT		Oral transit time
P		Plan
PAS		Penetration Aspiration Scale
PC		Presenting condition
PEG		Percutaneous endoscopic gastrostomy
PEJ		Percutaneous endoscopic jejunostomy
PMH		Past medical history
PT		Physiotherapist
PTT		Pharyngeal transit time
R		Right
RCSLT		Royal College of Speech and Language Therapists
RHR		Resting heart rate
RIG		Radiologically inserted gastrostomy
RR		Respiratory rate
Sats/O_2 sats/ SpO_2		Oxygen saturations
sEMG		Surface electromyography
SH		Social history
SLT		Speech and language therapist

SLTA	Speech and language therapy assistant
SMART	Specific, measurable, appropriate, realistic, timebound
SOL	Space-occupying lesion
SSRIs	Selective serotonin reuptake inhibitors
T/ temp	Temperature
TIA	Transient ischaemic attack
TOMs	Therapy Outcome Measures
TWST	Timed Water Swallow Test
UES	Upper esophageal sphincter
UMN	Upper motor neurone
VF	Videofluoroscopy
WCC	White cell count
WHO	World Health Organization
1/7	One day
1/52	One week

ACKNOWLEDGEMENTS

Thank you to my brilliant MSc Speech and Language Therapy students at Health Sciences University (HSU), Bournemouth, who gave me fantastic advice about what a student SLT or newly qualified practitioner might need from a book like this. The profession is in good hands.

Interdisciplinary working is so important in all aspects of client management. I would like to extend my thanks to all my HSU colleagues who contributed their profession-specific knowledge and expertise to the book – particularly Gráinne Ford, Dr Sherril Spencer, Louise Stanley and Parag Sawant.

Huge thanks to Fran Chandler and all the Milton Keynes Adult Speech and Language Therapy Service eating, drinking and swallowing clinicians, who so generously provided their top dysphagia tips – I hope I have done them all justice!

And finally, thanks to John, who constantly supports and encourages me to write, even though mostly he'd rather we were down at the beach.

INTRODUCTION

Assessing and managing the eating, drinking and swallowing (EDS) needs of our adult clients has become an increasingly important part of the speech and language therapist's (SLT) job. Students, newly qualified practitioners and those moving into this area of work from a different clinical caseload may lack confidence or feel ill-equipped to deal with what they face. EDS is often imbued with the lexicon of danger, risk and safety which can trouble the emergent practitioner. This text aims to bust the myth that EDS assessment and management is trickier than any other clinical area of SLT. Clinicians just need to be equipped with the right knowledge, tools, experience, support and confidence in order to thrive in this area and provide clients with the optimum care. The Royal College of Speech and Language Therapists' curriculum guidelines and competencies for newly qualified practitioners (2021) provide an essential framework to ensure that all SLTs can become safe, autonomous, competent and confident practitioners in EDS.

This book provides 50 top EDS tips based on my experience as a clinician, practice educator and lecturer, which will help you to navigate the sometimes choppy waters of EDS assessment and management, and steer you towards autonomy and competence in this exciting and rewarding clinical area.

The tips are arranged alphabetically to aid your navigation, forming an A-Z of EDS.

A IS FOR . . .

AETIOLOGIES

Understanding the aetiology (cause) of a client's EDS needs informs our clinical decision-making, including assessment strategy, management choice and client goals. Although each person will present differently and uniquely, patterns of difficulty may be evident depending on the underlying cause of the dysphagia (see also D for dysphagia). Hence, it is useful to have a working knowledge of the possible types of impairment related to the multifarious aetiologies. Causes of EDS needs in adults can broadly be divided into neurogenic, structural, functional and related to other issues (eg, physical and/or learning disability and ageing). Already you will be thinking that managing a functional swallowing difficulty will be very different from managing the swallowing symptoms of someone who has altered anatomy following head and neck surgery. When we discover the cause of the EDS need (from a referral, medical or other notes or a case history), we are already starting to make clinical decisions.

NEUROGENIC

As the etymology suggests, 'neuro-' (to do with the nervous system) '-genic' ('originating from') conditions affect either the central nervous system, the peripheral nervous system or both. If you look under N for neurological underpinnings and C for cranial nerves, you will see how intrinsic the nervous system is to the swallow process. It therefore stands to reason that a disruption to this system is likely to result in impairment to the swallow. Neurogenic aetiologies can further be divided into those conditions which occur abruptly and result in sudden-onset

EDS issues (eg, stroke or other brain injury), and those with a more gradual onset (eg, neurodegenerative conditions such as Parkinson's disease, motor neurone disease and Huntington's disease). The typical recovery trajectory in sudden-onset dysphagia is one of some spontaneous recovery, some recovery with therapeutic intervention and a plateauing of function. Intervention may include direct therapy techniques to improve function or temporary compensatory strategies. The trajectory in gradual-onset dysphagia is more one of steady (sometimes quite rapid) decline, with the aim of intervention being to maintain function for as long as possible, then to manage changes as they occur. Intervention in this case is less likely to be centred on improving function and more likely to focus on safer swallowing strategies and possibly preparing clients for enteral feeding (see under E). EDS needs in neurodegenerative conditions occur at different rates. For example, someone with Parkinson's disease may not experience dysphagia symptoms until they have been living with their diagnosis for several years, whereas dysphagia (and speech) signs may be the presenting issues in a client with motor neurone disease.

Some of the common patterns of impairment in neurogenic EDS can be seen in Table 1.

STRUCTURAL

Structural dysphagia can occur when a space-occupying lesion (SOL) or tumour disrupts the anatomy and therefore the physiology of the swallow. Tumours may occur anywhere along the aerodigestive tract, such as on the lips and tongue, in the pharynx or larynx, or deep in the floor of the mouth. The effect of the SOL will differ depending on both the site and size; some tumours will not impede the swallow at all.

Treatment for head and neck cancer almost always impacts the EDS process. Surgery will alter the anatomy – often quite radically – and in the immediate post-operative period there is swelling and pain. Patients who have undergone extensive surgery for head and neck cancer may have a tracheostomy tube inserted to aid their breathing (see under T) and may need to

Table 1 Common EDS issues related to various neurological conditions

Aetiology	Common EDS signs
Unilateral stroke	Weakness to the contralateral side (from the site of lesion) of the orofacial area (cranial nerve (CN) VII) and the tongue (CN XII) may impact oral manipulation of the bolus and containment of the bolus within the oral cavity, lip seal and intraoral pressure and anterior-posterior propulsion of the bolus. Unilateral weakness of the pharynx may hinder progression of the bolus. Unilateral weakness of velum may result in velopharyngeal incompetence. EDS signs are usually mild, often with complete recovery of function governed by CNs V, IX and X.
Brainstem stroke	Extensive difficulties if cranial nerves associated with swallowing (V, VII, IX, X, XII) are affected. May show flaccid signs (damage to cranial nerves) or spastic signs (because of damage to synapse with upper motor neurones). Oral preparatory and oral stages are characterised by reduced physical skills in general and limited movement of the articulators and the pharyngeal stage by reduced hyolaryngeal excursion and subsequent reduced opening of the cricopharyngeal sphincter (upper oesophageal sphincter).
Traumatic brain injury	Variable depending on site of lesion. Abnormal oral reflexes (eg, bruxism, bite reflex), recurrence of primitive reflexes seen in infancy (eg, suck-swallow and rooting). Possible presence of tracheostomy. Cognitive and behavioural issues may impact the safety of eating and drinking (eg, distractibility).
Dementia	Physical, cognitive and behavioural difficulties can all impact the different stages of the swallow. Prolonged oral preparatory stage with pocketing of food in the lateral sulci. Forgetting to eat or forgetting they have already eaten. Not recognising food (agnosia) or believing food is harmful. Not being able to sit at a table for a meal.

(*Continued*)

Table 1 (Continued)

Aetiology	Common EDS signs
Parkinson's disease	Anterior saliva escape. Reduced manipulation of the bolus and decreased mastication. Repetitive tongue-pumping. Slow oral transit time. Delay in triggering swallow reflex. Reduced airway protection. Piecemeal deglutition (multiple swallows on one bolus). Pharyngeal residue. Oesophageal obstruction. Reflux. Chest pain. Gastrointestinal dysfunction.
Motor neurone disease	Flaccidity/spasticity affecting manipulation and control of the bolus in the oral cavity. Reduced lip closure, resulting in anterior escape of saliva. Difficulties with anterior-posterior propulsion of the bolus. Flaccidity affecting velopharyngeal competence (closing off nasal cavity), with subsequent alteration to intraoral pressure and possible nasal regurgitation. Reduced laryngeal closure. Reduced breath support/weak cough/compromised airway.
Huntington's disease	Difficulty holding cutlery and cups. Constant choreic movement of limbs, making transport of food/fluid to mouth difficult. Problems with mastication and manipulation of the bolus in the oral cavity. Reduced lip closure. Difficulties with anterior-posterior propulsion of the bolus. Unpredictable inhalations. Postural instability, causing overspill of food/fluid into pharynx prior to swallow being triggered. Lack of coordination between oral and pharyngeal stages. Behavioural and cognitive issues. High energy needs in the context of reduced oral intake.

be nil by mouth (NBM) until the oedema (swelling) subsides and some healing occurs. Some surgery involves using flaps from elsewhere in the body to repair the area – for example, in glossectomy, the tongue might be repaired using a flap of skin from the radial forearm or bone from the fibula may be used to reconstruct the mandible. Flaps will not necessarily perform in the same way as the structure they have replaced. The SLT will monitor the client as healing occurs, with the aim of reintroducing oral intake if possible. Videofluoroscopy (VF) (an instrumental assessment technique using X-rays – see under V) may be useful to visualise the changed anatomy. Intervention may include advice on the most comfortable consistencies or safest head positions.

It can be quite shocking to see a patient on the ward directly after they have undergone radical head and neck surgery, especially if you are new to this clinical area. They may have large surgical wounds with stitches, clips and drains. Prepare yourself by asking a more experienced colleague what to expect.

During radiotherapy, although the X-rays are carefully targeted to the area of tumour using a bespoke mask-like structure, healthy tissue will inevitably get in the way and be damaged. Radiotherapy for head and neck cancer may therefore cause issues such as mucositis (inflammation of the mucosa of the mouth), fibrosis (stiffening) of tissue, trismus (tightened jaw muscles) and xerostomia (dry mouth), having an impact on the physiology of the swallow and the comfort and enjoyment of eating and drinking. Clients undergoing radiotherapy will need ongoing SLT monitoring for change to the swallow over time. The curative/palliative effects of radiotherapy, as well as the side effects, can last a few weeks after cessation of the treatment itself. Throughout the course of treatment (and beyond), swallowing may become acutely painful, necessitating texture modification and, in some cases, introduction of enteral feeding methods. As the side effects subside, the SLT will advise on the gradual reintroduction of oral intake.

If cancer of the larynx necessitates complete surgical removal of the larynx, the resultant new anatomy means that the trachea and oesophagus are no longer joined by a common structure (ie, the pharynx). In theory, this means that aspiration is impossible – all food and drink must enter the oesophagus and cannot inadvertently enter the trachea. However, the surgeon will usually create a fistula (hole) between the posterior tracheal and anterior oesophageal walls in order for a one-way valve or prosthesis to be sited, allowing the client to voice. This fistula may initially be plugged by a nasogastric tube (NGT) immediately postoperatively, keeping the hole patent while also providing a route for enteral feeding. Once the surgeon is confident that anastomosis (joining of tissue) has healed, they will liaise with the SLT, who can both site a valve for voicing and recommence oral intake. Despite the lack of a common structure between the trachea and the oesophagus with the new anatomical arrangement, there is nevertheless the potential for food/fluid/saliva to escape around the valve and into the airway if the valve is too small for the fistula, or if the one-way valve is failing for some reason (age of valve or build-up of candida albicans being common causes). Substances leaking into the trachea will obviously progress down into the lungs, so assiduous checking of the patency and fit of the valve is necessary – preferably by the client themselves, who is trained by the SLT to be alert to possible leakage. The client is advised to use a mirror with a good light source. They take a sip of an easily visible substance (milk is often used for this purpose) and watch for signs of milk seeping out around the edge of the valve. If leakage is detected by the client, they are advised to stop oral intake until the cause of the leak has been determined. Clients are also instructed by the SLT in how to clean and care for the valve to prolong its life and minimise the risk of leakage. A failing valve will need to be changed; some clients are trained to do this themselves, but others may need to see the SLT who can do this for them.

As an aside, if the valve becomes dislodged, a dilator or some tubing must be inserted into the fistula to prevent the hole from closing and needing to be surgically recreated. The fistula can close with remarkable alacrity (ie, within an hour).

When the larynx is removed and the anatomy is altered during surgery, the upper oesophageal sphincter no longer exists. This can lead to clients complaining of reflux as food and fluid come back up the oesophagus. Advice on positioning may be needed.

Clients with oesophageal cancer may experience problems with eating and drinking because of the tumour; squamous cell carcinomas normally present in the top part of the oesophagus and adenocarcinomas in the lower section. Dysphagia symptoms due to the SOL include chest pain and coughing, as food builds up above the level of the stricture (tumour) and may spill over into the laryngeal vestibule. As with head and neck cancer, treatment for oesophageal cancer may cause further dysphagic symptoms. For example, surgery often involves an incision in the anterior neck; if the recurrent laryngeal nerve (part of CN X, the vagus) is inadvertently damaged during the operation, the client may experience a weak cough and have reduced airway protection (as well as a weak voice, of course). Compensatory strategies such as head positions (chin tuck) and advice about avoiding some consistencies may be useful here.

During surgery, the cancerous part of the oesophagus is removed and the stomach pulled up into the chest and joined to the remaining oesophagus in a procedure called an 'oesophagectomy'. Sometimes the entire oesophagus has to be removed and the stomach brought right up and attached to the pharynx – this is referred to as a 'gastric pull-up'.

FUNCTIONAL

Some EDS symptoms may occur with no identifiable underlying structural or neurological cause and may therefore be termed 'functional'. Clients may demonstrate pre-disposing, precipitating and perpetuating factors in their lives, such as illness or stress. Functional dysphagia is normally oropharyngeal in nature, with symptoms including a reduced ability to control the bolus in the mouth (eg, anterior escape of the bolus) and an inability to trigger a swallow.

Despite the lack of underlying pathology, symptoms are nevertheless real for the client and can be highly distressing. As with any functional difficulty, treating functional EDS may involve a two-pronged clinical approach, employing both psychological and symptomatic therapy. For example, a client with the symptom of globus (the feeling of a lump in the throat) may benefit from therapy to challenge unhelpful thoughts (eg, cognitive behaviour therapy), alongside graded food trials (perhaps first using easily dissolved food, such as crisps or chocolate buttons).

AGEING

People who are ageing with no underlying neurological or structural pathologies may still experience some EDS issues. This is known as 'presbyphagia' – see under P for more information about this.

LEARNING DISABILITY AND PHYSICAL DISABILITY

Some people may not acquire their EDS needs through illness or accident – they may have dysphagia associated with a learning or physical disability from birth. Safety and enjoyment of eating and drinking for people with a learning disability may be affected by physical difficulties at any or all stages of the swallow, as well as behavioural and cognitive issues. Adults with a physical disability such as cerebral palsy may have movement problems which impact the swallow. For people with lifelong EDS needs, quality of life is paramount and should feature prominently in our management.

ANATOMY AND PHYSIOLOGY

Understanding the anatomy (structures) used in the swallow process is key to understanding the physiology (mechanism) and aids the clinical decision-making process. A good theoretical understanding of both the anatomy and physiology of the swallow is also important when we come to explain specific issues to clients or carers or train other professionals. You might want to practise drawing and labelling a diagram of the head and neck in the sagittal plane to ensure that you are totally familiar with the names of all the structures. Honing your drawing skills will also enable you to draw explanatory diagrams for clients and carers.

KEY STRUCTURES

Starting anteriorly, the key structures are as follows: lips, teeth, sulci (lateral and anterior), mandible, maxilla, tongue, hard palate, velum (soft palate), uvula, faucial arches, nasal cavity, nasopharynx, oropharynx, hypopharynx, epiglottis, hyoid bone, valleculae, pyriform sinuses (fossae), laryngeal vestibule, false vocal folds (vestibular folds), true vocal folds (cords), cricopharyngeal sphincter (upper oesophageal sphincter) and oesophagus.

Table 2 shows the different structures (in alphabetical order) and some key information about them.

Table 2 The anatomical structures involved in the swallow process with some key information

Structure	Key information
Cricopharyngeal sphincter	Also known as the upper oesophageal (or esophageal) sphincter (UES). This is closed until food/fluid approaches. Hyolaryngeal excursion contributes to UES opening.
Epiglottis	A leaf-shaped, cartilaginous structure. 'Epi' means 'above' (the glottis). Contributes to airway protection.
False vocal folds	Also called vestibular folds. Contribute to airway protection.
Faucial arches	If you look in someone's mouth, you will see the two arches with the uvula hanging down between them. The swallow reflex typically triggers when the head of the bolus touches the faucial arches. Pronounced /fɔsɪəl/
Hard palate	Made of bone, this constitutes the roof of the mouth.
Hyoid bone	A small, boomerang-shaped bone, attached to the tongue by the hyoglossus muscle, to the mandible by the suprahyoid muscles and to the larynx by the infrahyoid muscles.
Hypopharynx	The lowest part of the pharynx. Also called the 'laryngopharynx'.
Laryngeal vestibule	The area between the base of the epiglottis and the vestibular folds.

(*Continued*)

Table 2 (Continued)

Structure	Key information
Larynx	Comprised of the supraglottic, glottic and subglottic regions.
Lips	The adjective associated with the lips is 'labial'.
Mandible	Lower jaw (moveable).
Maxilla	Upper jaw (fixed).
Nasal cavity	Comprised of turbinates. The nasal cavity is closed off during swallowing by the velum meeting the posterior pharyngeal wall.
Nasopharynx	The top part of the pharynx.
Oesophagus	Comprised of striated muscle (top third), smooth muscle (lower third) and smooth and striated muscle (middle third).
Oropharynx	The mid part of the pharynx.
Pyriform sinuses	Also called the pyriform (pear-shaped) fossae. Small pockets in the hypopharynx.
Sulcus/sulci	The space between the inner cheeks and gum (lateral) and the lower lip and gum (anterior).
Teeth	Involved in biting and mastication.
Tongue	The adjectives associated with the tongue are 'lingual' or 'glossal'. Papillae covering the tongue contain tastebuds which can detect sweet, salty, sour, bitter and umami flavours. Only the anterior two-thirds (body) can be seen on examination. The posterior third (root or base) lies behind a slight groove called the 'sulcus terminalis'.
True vocal folds	Sometimes called 'vocal cords'. Important for airway protection.
Uvula	A small structure at the back of the mouth between the faucial arches. Means 'little grape'.
Valleculae	Small pockets in the oropharynx where the tongue meets the epiglottis.
Velum	Soft palate. Unlike the hard palate, the velum contains muscle and can move.

The respiratory tract and the digestive tract share the pharynx (divided into the nasopharynx, oropharynx and hypopharynx/laryngopharynx). The base of the pharynx divides into the larynx and trachea (a fixed, rigid, cartilaginous tube) and the oesophagus (a collapsed, muscular tube). Air flows freely through the trachea and the two bronchi and into the lungs. Food and fluid pass into the oesophagus via the cricopharyngeal sphincter, thereby dilating it. Regular muscular contraction of the oesophagus (peristalsis) pushes the food down. The lower oesophageal sphincter at the distal end of the oesophagus dilates to allow the food into stomach.

MUSCULATURE

The muscles involved in the EDS process are summarised in Table 3.

Table 3 The musculature involved in swallowing

Structure	Muscles	Involvement in swallow
Lower face and lips	Buccinator	Contracts to help contain food/fluid/saliva within the oral cavity. Contributes to intra-oral pressure.
	Orbicularis oris	Enables the lips to move and to close, so that food/fluid can be taken from a utensil or cup and held in the oral cavity. Lip seal also contributes to intra-oral pressure.
	Temporalis Masseter Pterygoids	Mastication (movement of the jaw).
Tongue	Intrinsic: vertical, transverse and longitudinal (inferior and superior). Extrinsic: genioglossus, hyoglossus, palatoglossus, styloglossus.	Fine movements needed in manipulation of the bolus and anterior-posterior transference of the bolus. Tongue base retraction. Elevation of lateral edge to facilitate bolus containment.
Velum	Tensor veli palatini Levator veli palatini Musculus uvulae Palatoglossus Palatopharyngeus	Soft palate elevation which closes off the nasal cavity.

(*Continued*)

Table 3 (Continued)

Structure	Muscles	Involvement in swallow
Pharynx	Superior pharyngeal constrictor Middle pharyngeal constrictor Inferior pharyngeal constrictor	Contract to push the bolus downwards towards the oesophagus.
Larynx	Extrinsic and intrinsic	Airway protection (see L for larynx for further details).

The muscles involved in swallowing are innervated by the cranial nerves, which in turn receive impulses from the upper motor neurones in the cortex. Sensory information from the various structures also travels along axons of the cranial nerves, synapse with sensory neurones in the brainstem and travel to the sensory cortex in the brain (for more details, see under N for neurological underpinnings).

PHYSIOLOGY

The swallow is typically described as being divided into four stages or phases. This is to enable the clinician to identify the point of difficulty and thereby devise a way to mitigate this. In reality, of course, all the stages are interlinked and an individual may have difficulties at more than one stage. Some clinicians and researchers lump the oral preparatory and oral stages together (calling this the 'oral stage'), but I prefer to separate them out for the purposes of pinpointing exactly where the breakdown is occurring.

ORAL PREPARATORY STAGE

Swallowing begins with the oral preparatory stage, which comprises physical, cognitive and sensory processes. Executive function in the brain enables us to decide whether we want to eat or not, judge whether we like a particular type of food or not and plan how big a mouthful we can manage. Fine and gross motor skills enable us to cut up, scoop or fork food or manipulate other utensils such as chopsticks. We are able to prepare the food into bite-sized portions and then transport it to our mouths. The cerebral cortex is alerted to the fact that swallowing is about to take place by these movements and through sensory input; we see, smell and touch food and drink. This stimulates production of saliva (in fact, even just thinking about food can do this). Opening the mouth (via movement of the mandible) enables food/fluid to enter the oral cavity and mastication (chewing) and manipulation of the food by the tongue take place, creating a cohesive mass known as a 'bolus'. Lip seal is not necessary at this stage from a physiologic point of view, although it is generally considered polite to close your mouth while chewing. Tension in the oral musculature, such as the buccinator, helps to keep the bolus in the oral cavity and prevents slippage into the space between the inner cheek and the gums, known as the lateral sulci. The oral preparatory stage is under voluntary control and lasts different lengths of time depending on the initial consistency of the food.

An example of an aetiology which may affect the oral preparatory stage is dementia; this stage may be prolonged, with clients pocketing food in the lateral sulci, or clients may show signs of not recognising food (agnosia).

ORAL STAGE

The oral stage is also under voluntary control and takes approximately one second, regardless of the initial consistency of the food. In this phase, the bolus is pushed from the front of the mouth to the back, ready for the swallow reflex to trigger as it reaches the faucial arches. This anterior-posterior transference of the bolus is sometimes referred to as a 'stripping motion' and entails the tip and then the blade of the tongue pressing against the hard palate, squeezing the bolus back as it does so. Lip seal *is* necessary during this stage, as well as buccal tension; closure of the mouth generates intra-oral pressure, which aids anterior-posterior transference and ensures that food or fluid does not exit anteriorly.

The time taken for the bolus to move from the front to the back of the mouth (ie, from commencement of the oral phase to the passing of the leading edge of the bolus across the point where the mandible crosses the tongue base) is known as the 'oral transit time' (OTT). The OTT may be measured objectively during VF.

An example of an aetiology which may affect the oral stage is unilateral stroke: weakness of one side of the tongue may impede the lingual stripping motion and unilateral weakness of the lips may mean that there is anterior escape of some of the bolus on that side.

PHARYNGEAL STAGE

At the point at which the head of the bolus contacts the faucial arches, the swallow reflex is triggered; the process is now no longer under voluntary control and is referred to as a 'reflex'. As the swallow triggers, the velum (soft palate) rises and meets the posterior pharyngeal wall, which in turn bulges slightly in an area known as 'Passavant's ridge' or 'pad'; this effectively seals off the nasal cavity, so that food and fluid are unable to enter, and intraoral and pharyngeal pressures are maintained. The larynx rises upwards and forwards (hyolaryngeal excursion), the vocal folds adduct (close) and the false vocal folds approximate. Because of this, breathing stops for a short while (apnoea) and the airway is protected from food/fluid entering. As the bolus enters the pharynx, the epiglottis is pushed down, providing further protection to the airway and directing the bolus towards the oesophagus in a chute-like fashion. As the larynx moves, the bolus makes contact with the upper oesophageal sphincter (also known as the 'cricopharyngeal sphincter'), causing it to relax and open to allow the bolus into the oesophagus.

The time taken from the point of swallow trigger to the bolus passing through the cricopharyngeal sphincter is known as the 'pharyngeal transit time' (PTT). The PTT may also be one of the measures taken during VF.

An example of an aetiology which may affect the pharyngeal stage is Parkinson's disease: the swallow reflex may be delayed, so that the bolus enters into the pharynx before it is triggered.

OESOPHAGEAL STAGE

The oesophageal stage comprises dilation of the oesophagus to accommodate the bolus and regular contractions of smooth muscle (peristalsis) which push the bolus through the oesophagus towards the lower oesophageal sphincter and the stomach.

An example of an aetiology which may affect the oesophageal stage is oesophageal cancer: a space-occupying lesion may occlude or partially occlude the oesophagus, thereby impeding peristalsis and progression of the bolus towards the stomach.

ASPIRATION, LARYNGEAL PENETRATION AND CHOKING

Aspiration is the progress of food, fluid or saliva into the trachea, past the level of the vocal folds. A cough is normally elicited; if there is no cough, this is known as 'silent aspiration'. Aspirated material continues along its path to the lungs; because of gravity and the fact that the right bronchus is comparatively more vertical than the left (which must accommodate the heart), aspirated material and/or the effects of aspiration can often be heard on auscultation (listening with a stethoscope) in the right basal lobe. When you are reviewing the medical notes, see whether the doctor has noted any crepitations or crackles in the right lower lobe of the lungs; sometimes this is denoted by a small diagram of the lungs with crosses to show where the crepitations have been heard. Crackles in the right lower lobe are suggestive of aspiration and should alert you to the possibility of dysphagia. The respiratory physiotherapist will also be able to listen to the chest and determine whether they hear any sounds possibly related to aspiration.

When you are carrying out a clinical swallow examination using oral trials or observing the client at a mealtime, look out for the following signs that may indicate that the client is aspirating:

- coughing (a cough may also indicate that the client is dealing successfully with laryngeal penetration);
- wet voice;
- eye-watering; or
- visible distress.

In your notes, you might state that the client is showing clinical signs of aspiration. This indicates that you suspect aspiration (through observation), but it is difficult to be definitive using subjective assessment strategies. For example, a client may experience laryngeal penetration but be able to cough and clear the airway; or they may experience laryngeal penetration, be able to cough but be unable to clear the airway of the bolus. Clinically, we are observing coughing but the two sequelae of the cough are very different. A clinical swallow examination (CSE) (with or without other methods such as cervical auscultation and pulse oximetry) can lead us to make an educated supposition about the likelihood that aspiration is occurring, but an instrumental assessment such as VF or fibreoptic endoscopic evaluation of swallowing (FEES) will allow us to give a definitive diagnosis. However, instrumental assessments may not be available or the client may be too unwell to tolerate them, so sometimes we have to rely on clinical observation and judgement.

Laryngeal penetration is when food, fluid or saliva enters the laryngeal vestibule but does not go past the level of the vocal folds into the trachea; the material is ejected back into the pharynx by coughing. Penetration of the laryngeal vestibule is common in people with or without dysphagia and, if the cough is working well, is not of major concern. However, in clients with a compromised airway, with a weak or even absent cough reflex, laryngeal penetration poses more of a problem, because the possibility of not ejecting and therefore aspirating the material is heightened.

Choking is when the trachea is completely occluded (blocked) by a foreign body. No air is able to enter the trachea and no air can be pushed out in order to dislodge the material. Sequelae of choking include anoxic brain injury (from reduced oxygen to the brain) and death; therefore, choking constitutes a medical emergency which needs immediate treatment in the form of stomach thrusts, for example. Make sure you familiarise yourself with local choking policies for your particular service or setting. Some foodstuffs which can constitute a choking hazard for clients at risk of aspiration include hard chunks of fruit and tough pieces of meat.

'Choking' is often mentioned in referrals, but more often than not the referrer means that they suspect the client is aspirating. I have received referrals in the past stating that the client is choking on water, but it is simply not possible for fluid to occlude the airway.

ASPIRATION PNEUMONIA

Not all aspiration will result in the client becoming unwell; some individuals aspirate habitually but never develop a chest infection. However, aspiration constitutes one of the risk factors for contracting aspiration pneumonia. The others include polypharmacy, poor oral hygiene, several underlying pre-existing pathologies, smoking and an underlying chest problem, such as chronic obstructive pulmonary disease (COPD) (Langmore et al, 1998).

It is not our role to diagnose aspiration pneumonia. However, our input to team discussions around findings from assessment may be an integral part of the diagnostic jigsaw. In the medical notes, we look out for any signs and symptoms which may indicate a chest infection, such as:

- productive cough;
- crackles/crepitations in the right lower lobe;
- high temperature (pyrexia); and
- raised white cell count.

A CLINICAL TOP TIP

You cannot definitively diagnose aspiration in a clinical evaluation of swallowing. If your clinical examination has led you to believe that aspiration of food and drink may be occurring, your notes should state: 'Clinical signs of aspiration noted.' Conversely, if your CSE leads you to believe that the person is not aspirating, your notes should state: 'No clinical signs of aspiration noted.'

Don't forget to consider silent aspiration if there are no clinical signs of aspiration but the person keeps developing chest infections.

B IS FOR . . .

BOLUS

During the oral preparatory stage, food is masticated (chewed), saliva is added and the tongue moves it around inside the oral cavity in a process known as oral manipulation. This results in the food transforming into a cohesive, moist ball, which is then referred to as a 'bolus' (from the Latin for 'ball'). In the oral stage, the bolus is transferred from the front to the back of the mouth by the tongue squeezing it against the hard palate towards the faucial arches ready to be swallowed. Different textures of food will take different lengths of time to be transformed into a bolus – a chunk of crusty bread will take much longer to chew than a ripe strawberry, for example. The bolus may not always remain as one mass: sometimes part of the bolus falls in the anterior and lateral sulci in the mouth; or a client may experience piecemeal deglutition, where the bolus splits and multiple swallows are needed to deal with it successfully.

The bolus may be manipulated for therapeutic reasons. For example, a cold (Kawakami et al, 2019), sour (Regan, 2020) or carbonated (Sdravou, Walshe and Dagdilelis, 2012) bolus is thought to heighten sensory input, thereby speeding up the swallow reflex. Have a look at a scoping review by Peña-Chávez et al (2023) for a full and detailed explanation of the different ways in which the bolus can be altered and the potential therapeutic effects on swallow physiology.

A client who has difficulty in chewing (eg, because of muscle weakness), has problems moving their tongue (eg, because of muscle weakness or surgery) or does not produce enough saliva (perhaps as a result of medication or radiotherapy) will therefore demonstrate more difficulty in forming a bolus. This may be counteracted by modifying textures and recommending International Dysphagia Diet Standardisation Initiative (IDDSI) Level 4 (puree), 5 (minced and moist), 6 (soft and bite-sized) or 7 (easy to chew). You may want to look at X for xerostomia for more details on the effects of xerostomia, sialorrhoea and changes to saliva viscosity on bolus formation.

Fluid boluses may also be thickened in an effort to slow down the oral and pharyngeal transit times, thereby lessening the chances of aspiration; but – as discussed under C for compensatory strategies – the evidence base for this is weak and the disadvantages of thickened fluid are manifold (Hansen et al, 2022).

BUCCINATOR, BUCCAL TENSION

The buccinator (from the Latin '*bucca*', meaning 'cheek') muscle of the lower face originates in both the maxilla and mandible and tautens during the oral preparatory and oral phases of the swallow so that:

- it is more difficult for food to fall into the space between the inner cheek and the gums (the lateral and anterior sulci);
- intra-oral (within the mouth) pressures are maintained;
- the bolus and saliva are kept within the oral cavity; and
- we are able to suck from a straw.

Movement of the buccinator is governed by the buccal branch of the facial nerve (CN VII). This lower branch of the facial nerve receives innervation from one side of the cerebral cortex only, so that unilateral damage to the cortex (eg, after a hemispheric stroke) can cause permanent weakness to the opposite side of the mouth to the lesion (ie, a right hemisphere stroke may cause a left-sided weakness to the buccinator).

You can test buccal tension during a cranial nerve (or oromotor) assessment by feeling the cheek, asking the client to puff out their cheeks with air or simply observing the swallow. As the orbicularis oris muscle is also innervated by CN VII, unilateral lip weakness and orofacial droop often co-occur with reduced buccal tension on the same side.

> **B CLINICAL TOP TIP**
>
> You can feel the buccinator by gently pressing just under the cheekbone (zygomatic bone) along the line of the upper teeth and along the line of the lower teeth, anteriorly-posteriorly.

C IS FOR . . .

CERVICAL AUSCULTATION

Often viewed as a supplement to the CSE, cervical auscultation employs a stethoscope to listen to sounds associated with the swallow, such as transfer of the bolus into the hypopharynx, post-swallow glottal release, pooling of food/fluid within the pharynx, return to normal breathing pattern post-swallow, exact number of swallows triggered and the opening of the cricopharyngeal (upper oesophageal) sphincter. Although evidence of its reliability as an assessment method has proved equivocal over the years since its inception, recent research has suggested its usefulness as a component of the SLT's assessment toolkit (Jaghbeer, Sutt and Bergström, 2023).

A stethoscope with a small bell and diaphragm (eg, those used in paediatrics) is placed onto the client's throat. The stethoscope is typically placed laterally, just above the cricoid cartilage. Earpieces should always face forwards and either the bell (for lower-frequency sounds) or the diaphragm side (for higher-frequency sounds) can be used. Don't forget to clean the bell/diaphragm and earpieces with an antiseptic wipe after use. Stethoscopes have become much more sensitive and reliable over the last few years (also with the functionality for recording sounds), perhaps leading to the greater perceived accuracy for swallow assessments mooted above.

As an assessment tool, cervical auscultation is relatively cheap, accessible and portable, and poses no risk to the client. It might be particularly useful for the clinician in the community who does not have easy access to more objective assessment methods such as VF and FEES. Cervical auscultation constitutes a useful addition to the assessment toolkit. However, dedicated training is recommended to be able to use cervical auscultation to its full potential to aid clinical reasoning and decision-making.

CLINICAL HISTORY

Before beginning the clinical swallow examination of the client, salient information must be gathered in order to structure and plan that assessment. We might view the entire assessment process like a jigsaw: information presented through clinical and case histories constitutes the initial two pieces and once this information has been reviewed, we can work out which assessment jigsaw pieces go next. For example, if the medical notes tell us that the client has a low level of arousal, our next assessment step might be observation only. If the medical notes tell us that the client is alert and obeying auditory commands, we may progress to the cranial nerve assessment (CNA).

Important and useful information can be gleaned through taking a thorough clinical history from the client's medical notes if these are available to the clinician. If full medical notes are not available (eg, if you are seeing a client in the community), some clinical information should be included in the initial referral.

SLTs need to be able to sift out the medical information from notes which may help them to make judgements about possible presentation, SLT diagnosis and further assessment choices.

Table 4 indicates what information might be useful and why.

Essentially, good information-gathering constitutes the beginning of the clinical decision-making process. For example, is the person's arousal level high enough to proceed with clinical assessment? Are they showing any signs of infection which could be suggestive of aspiration? What pattern of swallow difficulty might I expect, given the putative diagnosis? What is their swallow baseline, given their past medical history? Who is the significant other with whom I will need to make contact?

CLINICAL REASONING

As you progress through your pre-registration SLT course and into your first few years of practice, you will hone your clinical

Table 4 Information in medical notes important to the EDS clinician

Information	Abbreviation or shorthand used	Rationale
Date of admission		Indication of when the symptoms started.
Presenting condition	PC	Indication of possible or actual diagnosis.
	Notes may state 'imp', meaning the working diagnosis (or impression) – that is, before conclusive tests have been carried out.	
History of presenting condition	HPC	Helps with diagnosis.
Past medical history	PMH	Indication of pre-existing EDS needs.
		Indication of general health status prior to admission/prior to this episode.
Social history	SH	Tells us about the individual and their support network.
Drug history	DH	Some medications may impact the swallow (see M for medication).
On examination	O/E	Tells us how the client is presenting now.
Chest status	Diagram of the lungs with crepitations ('creps') or crackles marked with crosses.	If there is evidence of crepitations this may indicate aspiration, especially if in the right lower lobe.
Temperature	T/temp	Temperature of over normal (36.1–37.8 °C) is one of the indicators of infection (possibly chest). Sometimes the terms 'febrile'/'afebrile' or 'pyrexial'/'apyrexial' are used.

(*Continued*)

Table 4 (Continued)

Information	Abbreviation or shorthand used	Rationale
White cell count	WCC/ ↑WCC	Raised white cell count may be an indicator of infection.
Heart rate	HR/RHR (resting heart rate) bpm (beats per minute).	High resting heart rate may indicate infection.
Oxygen saturation level	Sats/O_2 sats/SpO_2	Reduced oxygen saturations may indicate respiratory difficulties (see also P for pulse oximetry).
Respiratory rate	RR	Increased respiratory rate may indicate a compromised chest.
Cranial nerve assessment	CNA/ CN Ax	Although the SLT will carry out an EDS-specific CNA, this gives a summary of the functioning of all 12 cranial nerves.
Glasgow Coma Scale	GCS (score /15, divided into eyes (E), verbal response (V) and motor response (M))	Tells us about the client's arousal level.
Plan	P	Next steps: referrals to other multi-disciplinary team (MDT) members; investigations (eg, X-rays, scans and blood tests); when the doctor plans to review.

reasoning skills. As an autonomous practitioner, an SLT must make good clinical decisions based on sound rationale, rooted in the evidence base. The following hypothetical case studies are designed to help you practise your clinical reasoning and clinical decision-making skills. Work through them either alone or with a colleague and compare your decisions with mine in the appendix. Really explore and justify your rationale for each decision.

JUDITH

Judith (54) had a right hemisphere stroke three days ago. A CT scan shows evidence of ischaemic damage in the right frontotemporal area. She was drowsy for the first two days but is now alert and talking. Judith is right-handed. The medical team have requested a swallow assessment.

The latest entry in the medical notes states the following:

PC: right hemisphere ischaemic stroke (frontotemporal)
HPC: 1/52 history of TIAs – seen in TIA clinic
PMH: hypertension, hiatus hernia
DH: omeprazole
SH: works as TA in a primary school, lives alone
O/E
Pt admitted 3 days ago with suspected right hemisphere stroke – confirmed by CT
Fully alert and talking in sentences – dysarthria in evidence.
Left-sided hemiparesis. Able to transfer from bed to chair with assistance of one.
Chest clear – no creps heard on auscultation.
Apyrexial - temp: 36.7°C
No raised WCC
Sats 100%
Currently NBM – IV fluids.
P: refer to SLT for swallow and speech

Your initial SLT EDS assessment shows the following: (table 5)
What is your SLT diagnosis?
What are your next steps?

Table 5 Results of Judith's CSE

CNA	V: Good mouth opening, slightly reduced strength left side of jaw. VII: Reduced range and strength of movement of lips on left, air/saliva escape left side. X: Strong volitional cough, voicing clear, soft palate symmetrical on /ɑ/. XII: Reduced range of movement and reduced strength left side of tongue, reduced rate of lateral movement, tongue deviates to left on protrusion.
Laryngeal palpation	Good forward and upward movement of the larynx felt. Prompt dry swallow.
Oral trials	Trial 1 (water from spoon): Anterior escape of water, prompt swallow, throat-clear post-swallow. Trial 2 (water from cup): anterior escape of water, prompt swallow, cough post-swallow. Trial 3 (IDDSI Level 2 – thickened squash from cup): no anterior escape of the bolus, prompt swallow elicited. No cough. Voice clear post-swallow. Trial 4 (IDDSI Level 1): As above Trial 5 (IDDSI Level 4 – yoghurt): No anterior escape of bolus, prompt swallow elicited. No cough. Voice clear post-swallow. Trial 6 (IDDSI Level 4 – yoghurt): As above.

PRAKASH

Prakash (62) had a brainstem stroke 14 days ago. He was initially very drowsy and kept nil by mouth. He now presents with a GCS score of 13/15 (E=4, V=3, M=6). Prakash can understand what is said to him; however, he has minimal residual speech. He communicates very proficiently by using an E-Tran frame. Nursing staff decided not to carry out a swallow screen, as oral movements were minimal.

The latest entry in the medical notes states the following:

PC: Brainstem stroke (CT scan shows large infarct extending into pons and medulla).
HPC: Patient complaining of feeling unwell for 1 day prior to admission. Collapsed at home.

PMH: Hypertension, NIDDM, depression and anxiety, asthma.
DH: Fluoxetine, lisinopril, salbutamol.
SH: Lives with wife, 2 adult sons live nearby, retired supermarket manager.
O/E
Pt admitted 14 days ago. GCS on admission 9/15 (E=3, V=1, M=5) – now 13/15.
Vocalising but unable to produce recognisable words. Seems to understand? Labile.
Unable to move ULs/ LLs – some movement in head. In profiling bed – needs hoist to transfer from bed to chair.
NBM with NGT in situ.
CN exam not carried out but pt able to move eyes up and down and laterally.
Chest clear – no creps heard on auscultation.
Apyrexial – temp: 37°C.
No raised WCC.
Sats 98%.
P:

- Refer to SLT for swallow assessment.
- Refer to dietitian.
- Refer to physio/ OT for wheelchair assessment.
- R/v in 1/7.

What are the salient pieces of information and what do they tell you?

Now that you have completed a clinical history, it's time to move on to the case history. What questions do you want to ask Prakash and his wife, Meera?

Once you have thought about this, move on to the next section, which shows Prakash and Meera's answers to the SLT's questions. Prakash can indicate 'yes' and 'no' by looking up and down respectively, and can convey some novel messages using the E-Tran frame.

Prakash then becomes visibly upset, so the conversation is terminated.

Table 6 Questions asked by the SLT in taking the case history and Meera and Prakash's responses

SLT	Meera	Prakash
Can you tell me a bit about what has happened to you?	Been in hospital for 14 days – admitted by ambulance after collapsing at home. Doctors have informed them that Prakash has had a brainstem stroke.	
Did you have any difficulties with eating and drinking prior to this?	No – nothing.	Looks down for no.
Do you have any pain when you swallow?		Looks down for no.
Have you had any chest problems since you came into hospital?	Explains that he had a short course of antibiotics shortly after admission, but these have now stopped and so has the coughing.	Looks up for yes.
Did you have problems with breathing or coughing before you came into hospital?		Prakash indicates yes and spells out 'inhaler' on E-Tran frame.
Is there anything you want to ask me?	Meera explains that they do not eat meat, eggs or fish for religious reasons.	Indicates 'no meat' using the E-Tran frame. Spells out 'food when . . .'

What further information have you gathered from the case history?

You now carry out a clinical swallow examination – here are the results:

ORAL HYGIENE EXAM

- Dry saliva around lips and adhering to hard palate.
- White patches on tongue.

CNA

Table 7 Results of Prakash's CNA

Cranial nerve	Results
V Trigeminal	Reduced mouth-opening. Weak movement against resistance. Poor lateral jaw movement. Intra-oral and peri-oral sensation not assessed.
VII Facial	Lips symmetrical at rest, low tone. Approximation of /i/ and /u/ but slow. Anterior escape of saliva in evidence. Air escape noted via lips when client asked to puff up cheeks.
X Vagus	Soft palate looks symmetrical at rest – client able to produce weak /ɑ/. Some nasal escape noted when client asked to puff up cheeks. Able to cough to command – reduced strength.
XII Hypoglossal	Tongue symmetrical and flaccid at rest. Fasciculations noted. Reduced ability to protrude tongue and move tongue laterally. Unable to push tongue into cheek; unable to lick lips.

LARYNGEAL PALPATION

Laryngeal palpation showed reduced hyolaryngeal excursion with suspected prolonged oral-prep and oral stages.

ORAL TRIALS

1st bolus: 1 x teaspoon smooth yoghurt:

- Opened mouth slightly to approach of spoon.
- Prolonged oral preparatory stage with ++ tongue-pumping and some anterior escape.
- Swallow elicited – cough post-swallow.
- No oral residue noted but difficult to see into mouth because of reduced mouth-opening.

2nd bolus: 1 x teaspoon smooth yoghurt:

- Opened mouth slightly to approach of spoon.
- Prolonged oral preparatory stage with ++ tongue-pumping and some anterior escape.

- Swallow elicited – no cough post-swallow.
- No oral residue noted but difficult to see into mouth because of reduced mouth-opening.

Sats dropped from 98% to 94% after swallow trials.
Can you start to draw any conclusions from the CSE?
What are your next steps?

TOMMY

Tommy (51) is currently undergoing a course of radiotherapy for cancer (T1 N0 M0) of the left parotid salivary gland. During his second week of treatment (of seven), he is seen jointly by you as the SLT and the dietitian.

Tommy is complaining of the following:

- reduced saliva/dry mouth;
- pain on swallowing;
- reduced mouth-opening;
- effortful swallowing;
- loss of enjoyment of eating and drinking; and
- weight loss.

What are your next steps in managing Tommy's EDS needs?

DERVLA

Dervla was diagnosed with motor neurone disease 12 months ago. She is experiencing changes to her speech and to her EDS, including:

- reduced breath support with a weak cough;
- slow tongue movements;
- delayed swallow reflex; and
- occasional coughing on some consistencies.

She has had no chest infections.
How will these issues affect the safety of her swallow and enjoyment of eating and drinking?

What might management of Dervla look like in the next few months?

Have a look at the appendix for indicative answers to the clinical scenarios – do you agree?

CLINICAL SWALLOW EXAMINATION (CSE)

The CSE – sometimes referred to as the 'bedside assessment' or simply 'clinical exam' – is carried out by the SLT after information has been gathered from clinical notes and a case history. The CSE comprises four main elements:

- observation;
- CNA (see below);
- laryngeal palpation (see under L); and
- oral trials.

Some therapists also include the use of cervical auscultation in their CSE.

Observation of the client can tell us a number of things – and, indeed, this may be the only aspect of the CSE that we are able to carry out for a client with a low arousal level, or someone who is supine and cannot be repositioned, for example. We can look for spontaneous swallows and saliva control, orofacial symmetry, breathing pattern, vocal quality, any abnormal oral reflexes and general oral hygiene.

The CNA is described below and laryngeal palpation is described under L for larynx.

Based on the results of observation, the CNA and laryngeal palpation, the clinician may attempt some oral trials to assess the likelihood of aspiration on oral intake. Table 8 shows examples of this type of clinical decision-making.

If you are an SLT on a ward, ensure that some appropriate foodstuffs are always available, such as yoghurts and bananas. If you are seeing a client in their own home, phone them beforehand so that they can supply food of varying consistencies.

The results of the CSE may enable the clinician to draw up person-centred goals and an intervention plan; or they may lead

Table 8 Rationale for oral trials

Result from observation, CNA and/or laryngeal palpation	Oral trial (bolus type)	Rationale
Absent/very reduced oral movements	None.	Inability to manipulate or control bolus. Risk of aspiration pre-swallow.
Mild/moderate lip weakness	IDDSI Level 1 fluids. IDDSI Level 2 fluids. IDDSI Level 4 food.	Difficulty holding fluid in the mouth. Reduced intra-oral pressure.
Mild/moderate reduction in tongue movements	IDDSI Level 1 fluids. IDDSI Level 2 fluids. IDDSI Level 4 food.	Difficulty manipulating/controlling the bolus.
Mild/moderate reduction in lateral jaw movement (mastication)	IDDSI Levels 4, 5, 6.	Difficulty in chewing a solid bolus.
Reduced laryngeal excursion	Water. No solids.	Possible reduction in airway protection – aspirated water causes fewer problems than water with thickener or food. Possible reduced cricopharyngeal opening.

the clinician to want to gain further details about the swallow which can only be achieved through the use of instrumental assessment techniques such as VF or FEES.

COMPENSATORY STRATEGIES

In contrast to direct therapy techniques, compensatory strategies aim not to improve swallow physiology but rather to alter swallow physiology temporarily by manipulating the anatomy or the bolus, thereby minimising the risk of aspiration.

HEAD/BODY POSITIONING

The optimal position for safe swallowing is upright with the head, neck and trunk in midline. However, altering head position subtly (but often very effectively) changes the anatomy and can render the swallow safer. For example, tucking the chin down towards the chest effectively widens the valleculae and narrows the entrance to the laryngeal vestibule. This therefore may be a useful technique for a client with reduced airway protection and/or a delay in swallow trigger. Common head positions used in clinical practice are listed in Table 9.

The key advantages of head/body positioning as a compensatory strategy are that they may have less impact on quality of life than other strategies (eg, texture modification), and they may be very useful temporary measures when the EDS landscape is changing quite rapidly (eg, for people entering the last weeks and days of life).

Disadvantages may be that the head/body positions seem unnatural to the client – they may have difficulty remembering to implement them or feel self-conscious in a social eating environment. Judicious use of VF as a biofeedback tool may be merited here; if the client can see the benefit of a head position, they are far more likely to implement it. Other simple strategies may be introduced to help the client to remember head positions, such as words/diagrams on a placemat or the client's wheelchair tray.

Table 9 Head/body positions with rationale

Head/body position	Rationale	Recommended for
Chin tuck	Minimises airway opening and maximises entrance to oesophagus.	Reduced airway protection. Delayed swallow trigger.
Head turn (to the affected side)	Closes off one side of pharynx – encourages the bolus down the stronger side.	Unilateral pharyngeal weakness.
Head tilt (to the stronger side)	Encourages the bolus down the stronger side of the pharynx.	Unilateral pharyngeal weakness.
Semi-reclined	Gravity helps with anterior-posterior movement of the bolus.	Reduced oral phase abilities (eg after partial glossectomy) in the context of good pharyngeal phase and airway protection.

SWALLOW MANOEUVRES

Encouraging the client to swallow in a slightly modified way may also be protective. Swallow manoeuvres were first advocated by Logemann (1996) and are predicated on the client having good cognitive skills and the ability to understand both the

Table 10 Common swallow manoeuvres with rationale.

Manoeuvre	Instructions to client	Rationale	Good for
Effortful	'As you swallow, squeeze your tongue and throat muscles as tightly as you can.'	Increases pharyngeal pressure and reduces pharyngeal residue.	People with pharyngeal residue post-swallow.
Mendelsohn	'As you are about to swallow, feel your voicebox/larynx rise up. Hold this position, then swallow.'	Improves hyolaryngeal excursion and airway protection.	People with reduced airway protection (eg, weak cough).
Supraglottic	'Just before you swallow, take a breath and hold. Swallow. Cough or huff immediately after you have swallowed. Breathe out.'	Clears pharynx of residue.	People with post-swallow pharyngeal residue.
Super-supraglottic	'Hold your breath tightly and bear down, as if you were lifting something heavy or were straining. Swallow with effort, squeezing your tongue and throat muscles. Cough immediately after swallowing and breathe out.'	Protects airway. Increases pressure. Clears residue.	People with reduced airway protection/reduced pharyngeal constriction, pharyngeal residue.

instructions and the rationale. Keep the instructions succinct and provide them in written format too. Some SLTs provide a video of how to carry out the manoeuvre. As for head positions, the client may find it difficult to remember swallow manoeuvres or feel socially embarrassed to implement them during mealtimes; VF may again be useful in order for both you and the client to view the efficacy of this approach. Discussion with you about how manoeuvres impact the swallow positively may also be a motivational force.

CHANGES TO THE ENVIRONMENT

Simple changes to the environment may make for safer eating and drinking. For example, a client with a head injury who is easily distracted may benefit from eating in a quiet room with no other diners or noise, such as the television or radio, in the background. A familiar dining room may help a person with dementia to recognise mealtimes; however, it is worth remembering that some people with dementia will find it difficult to remain seated for a length of time and may prefer to eat smaller meals at more regular intervals. Lunchtime assessments are always a useful tool for ascertaining what changes to the environment may benefit the client and make eating and drinking safer and more enjoyable.

HELPING THE PERSON TO EAT AND DRINK

Although being helped to eat and drink by someone else effectively bypasses some of the oral preparatory stage and can have a detrimental effect on that phase of the swallow, assisting someone may also bring some compensatory benefits. For example, consider a patient who has a right-sided hemianopia: if the helper sits to their left, visual stimulus of the food will be enhanced. Similarly, a helper can supplement the oral preparatory stage by describing the food to a person who is visually impaired or who has significant cognitive issues.

Helping someone else to eat and drink is important work and part of your role may be to encourage and train people who undertake this. Formal training sessions as well as observation of mealtimes will enable you to give advice and guidance for assisting specific clients. General guidance may include the following:

- Check the SLT's recommendations before the meal.
- If the client has thickened fluids, follow the manufacturer's instructions. Some thickened drinks become even thicker if left for long periods of time, or an enzyme in saliva (amylase) may cause the fluid to separate.
- Check that the client understands any recommended head positions or manoeuvres.
- Ask the client (or their carer) what their preferred utensils are.
- Ask the client whether they prefer a spoonful of one foodstuff or multiple tastes on one spoon.
- Avoid mixing up food on the plate. IDDSI Level 4/5 food can look particularly unappetising when all mixed up together.
- Look for the swallow – you should see the voice box rise up and down. Don't introduce the next spoonful until you have seen a swallow.
- Try to avoid talking/laughing during mealtimes – save your conversation for between courses or after the meal, so that the person is not tempted to talk or laugh with food in their mouth.
- Give the client plenty of time.
- Ensure that you are aware of local procedures in the event of choking.

UTENSILS

Enabling the client to eat and drink independently is desirable not only from a dignity and enjoyment perspective but also from a physiological one – the cortex is better prepared for the act of swallowing if oral preparatory steps such as moving the food or the cup to the mouth are implemented. Utensils which facilitate independence should therefore always be considered and joint-working with the occupational therapist (OT) can help us to select the best adaptive cutlery and crockery. For example, a cup with a cutaway edge enables the client to finish a drink without the need to tip the head back; a heated plate ensures that a meal stays hot for longer if eating is slow; and cutlery with specialised handles may allow someone with limited fine motor skills to continue to bring food to their mouth. You could consider a spoon with a shallow bowl for people with reduced mouth-opening; however, try to avoid using utensils which are designed for babies and children.

TEXTURE MODIFICATION

The consistency of food may be modified to render the swallow process safer and more enjoyable for the individual. For example, someone who has reduced lateral jaw movement (and therefore reduced mastication) and poor tongue movement (and therefore poor manipulation and control of the bolus in the oral cavity) may benefit from a softer texture, such as IDDSI Level 4 or 5. Try to keep textures as close to normal as possible (eg, recommend foods that are naturally minced and moist, such as shepherd's pie for Level 5). Always dissuade relatives from offering baby foods, however well intentioned.

Modification of fluids is more contentious and the evidence base is weak. However, it might still be necessary to thicken fluids for some clients in order to slow down the oral and pharyngeal transit times of the bolus. Thickened fluids are often not thirst-quenching or particularly palatable, so they should be recommended with circumspection and the clinical need for them should be constantly re-evaluated. Various proprietary thickening agents are available and often an SLT service will use a particular one. It is worth checking for new products as they come on the market. Currently, thickening agents must be prescribed by a medical doctor, so you will have to liaise with the general practitioner (GP) in the community or the doctor in the hospital if you feel that modified fluids are merited.

See under I for IDDSI for more about consistencies.

CRANIAL NERVES, CRANIAL NERVE ASSESSMENT (CNA)

There are 12 pairs of cranial nerves, which form part of the peripheral nervous system. Neurones from the motor and sensory cortices of the brain synapse with the cranial nerves and from here messages are conveyed to the muscle end plate and from sensory receptors in skin and mucosa. Smell, sight and head position are governed by CNs I, II and XI respectively, but the main cranial nerves involved in EDS are V trigeminal, VII facial, IX glossopharyngeal, X vagal and XII hypoglossal (by convention, the cranial nerves are always denoted with Roman numerals).

These cranial nerves originate in the brainstem (V and VII from the pons and IX, X and XII from the medulla), where they synapse with the upper motor/sensory neurones coming from/to the motor and sensory cortices in the brain. All the cranial nerves are bilaterally innervated by the upper motor neurones, except for the lower branch of VII and all of XII. These two cranial nerves receive innervation from one side only; if that side is damaged – through a stroke, for example – the other side is unable to compensate and permanent damage to function may occur. To illustrate this, someone who has had a left hemisphere stroke may show residual orofacial weakness on the right and a tongue which deviates to the right on protrusion (the stronger side of the tongue pushes the weaker side across the midline). However, the same patient may have symmetrical, normal movement to the jaw, upper face and velum (because CN V, the upper branches of CN VII and CN X are bilaterally innervated). However, it may take a few hours for the other side to compensate, so clients seen immediately after the stroke has occurred may show unilateral weakness of the upper face, jaw and soft palate. It is also not uncommon for this bilaterality to be uneven so that some residual weakness may remain.

Table 11 shows how these cranial nerves are involved in the EDS process.

See under N for more information about the neurological underpinnings of the swallow process.

The cranial nerves in numerical order provide a useful framework for assessing the movement of and sensation in the structures associated with swallowing. The CNA (sometimes referred to as an 'oromotor assessment' or 'oral exam') comprises part of the CSE (along with observation, laryngeal palpation and oral trials).

Table 11 The five main cranial nerves involved in the swallowing process

Cranial nerve	Sensory involvement	Motor involvement
V trigeminal	Face, around mouth, inside mouth.	Muscles of mastication, opening and closing of jaw.
VII facial	Taste anterior two-thirds of tongue.	Lip closure. Lip movement. Buccal tension.
IX glossopharyngeal	Taste posterior one-third of tongue.	Stylopharyngeus muscle (dilates the pharynx). Elevation of larynx and pharynx.
X vagus	Larynx (cough). Pharynx.	Palatoglossus muscle (raises the back of the tongue). Pharyngeal constrictors. Movement of soft palate. Closure of the vocal folds.
XII hypoglossal	None.	Movement of all intrinsic muscles of tongue. Movement of all extrinsic muscles of tongue (bar the palatoglossus).

To carry out a CNA, you will need a pen torch, a tongue depressor and gloves. Essentially, you are looking for:

- sensation (V, VII, X);
- range of movement (V, VII, XII);
- rate of movement (V, VII, XII);
- strength of movement (V, VII, X, XII); and
- symmetry (V, VII, X, XII).

Table 12 offers a framework on which to base your CNA and table 13 presents a simplified format to use with a client.

You will notice that although CN IX is important in the swallow process, as it is involved in the triggering of the swallow reflex and in constriction and dilation of the pharynx, these are difficult aspects to assess clinically. CN IX also governs the gag reflex and some doctors may test for this; however, most SLTs will not

Table 12 Assessing the cranial nerves

Cranial nerve	How?	Instruction	What?	Why?
V Trigeminal	Open/close mouth.	'Can you open and close your mouth? Now do that as fast as you can.'	Range and speed of movement.	Mouth-opening.
	Apply gentle pressure to jaw – can client resist pressure?	'I'm going to push gently on your jaw – try to keep your mouth open.'	Strength of movement.	Strength of movement for mouth-opening and mastication.
	Lateral jaw movement.	'Can you move your jaw from side to side?'	Range of movement.	Mastication.
	Touch the blade of the tongue with a (moistened) tongue depressor: step back from the tip posteriorly.	'I'm going to touch the blade of your tongue with a tongue depressor – can you feel this?'	Intra-oral sensation.	Awareness of bolus in the mouth.
	Touch around the mouth with a tongue depressor.	'Close your eyes. Point to where I touch you.'	Peri-oral sensation.	Awareness of bolus in the mouth.

(*Continued*)

Table 12 (Continued)

Cranial nerve	How?	Instruction	What?	Why?
VII Facial	Look for symmetry of lips at rest and on /i/ and /u/.	'Say /u/ and /i/ – now do this as fast as you can.'	Symmetry or asymmetry, range and speed of movement.	Helps to distinguish between unilateral or bilateral weakness. Range and speed of movement may affect ability to take food/fluid from spoon/cup.
	Look for anterior escape of saliva.		Lip seal.	
	Puff up cheeks – check for air escape (oral/nasal).	'Puff up your cheeks with air. Hold the air in your mouth for a few seconds. Now release.'	Lip seal.	Reduced lip seal would affect the ability to keep bolus in the oral cavity and intra-oral pressure.

(*Continued*)

Table 12 (Continued)

Cranial nerve	How?	Instruction	What?	Why?
X Vagus	Look at soft palate at rest and on /ɑ/. Press down on the tongue blade with a tongue depressor; use a torch.	'Open your mouth and say /ɑ/.'	Symmetry of soft palate at rest and when raised.	Lack of symmetry may indicate unilateral weakness and therefore reduced velopharyngeal competence.
	Puff up cheeks: listen for nasal escape.	'Puff up your cheeks with air. Hold the air in your mouth for a few seconds. Now release.'	Velopharyngeal competence.	Lack of velopharyngeal competence could lead to reduced intra-oral pressure and nasal regurgitation.
	Laryngeal palpation.	'I'm going to place my fingers gently on your throat – now swallow.'	Laryngeal movement.	Airway protection, timing of swallow, cricopharyngeal/upper oesophageal sphincter opening.
	Vocal quality.	'Can you clear your throat/cough?'	Vocal fold adduction. Food/fluid/saliva in laryngeal vestibule.	Airway protection.

(*Continued*)

Table 12 (Continued)

Cranial nerve	How?	Instruction	What?	Why?
XII Hypoglossal	Look at the tongue at rest.	'Open your mouth.'	Symmetry, asymmetry, fasciculations, atrophy.	Helps to distinguish between upper motor neurone and lower motor neurone involvement.
	Tongue protrusion.	'Stick out your tongue.'	Deviation from midline.	Unilateral upper motor neurone issue.
	Lateral tongue movement.	'Move your tongue from side to side. Now do that as quickly as you can.'	Range, strength and rate of movement.	Bolus manipulation.
	Tongue strength against gloved finger.	'Push your tongue into your cheek and press against my finger as hard as you can.'	Strength and range of movement.	Anterior posterior movement of bolus. Lingual manipulation of bolus.
	Range of tongue movement.	'Lick all the way around your lips.'	Range of movement.	Ability to clear oral residue.

Table 13 Simplified CNA

Cranial nerve	Instruction	Comments
V	'Open/ close your mouth.' 'Keep your mouth open as I press up gently on your jaw.' 'Move your jaw from side to side.' 'Can you feel this?' (Moistened tongue depressor stepped along blade of tongue.) 'Close your eyes and point to where I touch you.' (Around mouth.)	
VII	(Look for symmetry and saliva escape at rest.) 'Say /u/ and /i/. Do that five times. Now do that as fast as you can.' 'Puff up your cheeks with air. Hold the air in your mouth for a few seconds. Now release.' (Look for oral (lip seal) and nasal (velopharyngeal competence) escape of air.)	
X	'Open your mouth and say /ɑ/.' 'I'm going to place my fingers gently just under your chin – now swallow.' 'Can you clear your throat/cough?'	
XII	'Open your mouth.' 'Stick out your tongue.' 'Move your tongue from side to side. Now do that as fast as you can.' 'Lick all the way around your lips.' 'Push your tongue into your cheek and press against my finger as hard as you can.'	

because not only is the efficacy of the gag irrelevant to the efficacy of the swallow, but testing the gag is highly unpleasant and the antithesis of therapeutic.

The results of a CNA should lead us onto the next step, which is usually trials of food and fluids (see above). If the client's cranial nerves and the associated movement/sensation are severely affected, we would not proceed with oral trials. Instead, our management might take the form of watchful waiting (assessment may have taken place soon post-onset and some spontaneous neurological recovery is expected), or perhaps a programme of direct therapy which does not involve oral intake, such as oromotor exercises.

Although a CNA is useful, it may not be possible or desirable to carry it out for some clients – for example, a client who is unable to follow instructions because of cognitive and/or language difficulties, a client with severe non-verbal oral apraxia or a client with a low level of arousal.

> **C CLINICAL TOP TIP**
>
> Hone your clinical reasoning skills: what does it mean in terms of the swallow if a cranial nerve is affected? It's fine to take a form such as the one above in with you when you assess your client to help you remember all the steps of a CNA.

D IS FOR . . .

DENTITION

An adult human has 32 teeth, comprising incisors (which, as the name suggests, are used for cutting), canines (which tear food), and premolars and molars (which crush and grind food). The tearing and crushing functions are particularly useful in the oral preparatory stage of the swallow, when food is being formed into a bolus during mastication.

Being edentulous (ie, not having teeth) will impact an individual's ability to chew and form a bolus. Older clients may have a partial or full denture – ensure that this is in situ before conducting a CSE! Sometimes dentures become ill-fitting following illness, as soft tissue may become depleted; a reassessment by a dentist may be merited.

Individuals undergoing radiotherapy to the head and neck because of a cancer diagnosis may have preventative or prophylactic tooth extraction. This is because radiation may attack the blood vessels leading to the teeth, causing irreparable damage to blood supply and subsequent death and decay of the tooth. Any decay in the oral cavity may result in bacteria entering the bloodstream or the lungs if aspirated. People suffering from mucositis as a result of radiotherapy may find oral hygiene difficult to maintain because of significant pain, which puts them at risk of tooth cavities. Reduction in saliva may mean that food debris is not washed away as readily and that acidic environments are not neutralised. If radiotherapy patients require tooth extraction because of cavities, there is the risk of developing necrosis of the mandible/maxilla as a result of reduced blood flow and therefore oxygen supply (osteoradionecrosis) to the area.

DOI: 10.4324/9781003480877-4

The NHS recommends toothbrushing twice a day for about two minutes with a fluoride toothpaste to maintain good teeth and gum health. See under O for how good oral hygiene might be maintained for people with EDS needs and how oral care might be provided for those who are unable to carry this out for themselves.

DIRECT THERAPY TECHNIQUES

In contrast to compensatory techniques (see C), the aim of direct EDS therapy is to improve swallow physiology, thereby minimising aspiration and maximising safety. As with all therapeutic intervention, it is your job as the clinician to analyse the assessment results and decide on the best technique for any given client and presentation. Tables 14 and 15 show some therapy techniques which address the different stages of the swallow.

Direct therapy techniques may constitute the intervention which helps the client get from their baseline to their target goal. You may want to combine direct therapy approaches which target the physiological impairment with other management which may compensate for the impairment or with interventions that address quality of life.

DYSPHAGIA

Dysphagia (from the Greek '*dys*', denoting 'something wrong with', and '*phagein*', meaning 'to eat') results when there is disruption to the swallow process. The aetiologies which may lead to dysphagia are discussed under A. If a person has dysphagia, they may have difficulties at any or all of the different stages of the swallow process and may be at risk of aspiration before, during or after the swallow.

Table 16 shows examples of some dysphagia symptoms at each of the four stages of the swallow.

In recent years, SLTs have tended to refer to 'EDS needs' rather than 'dysphagia'. There are several reasons why 'EDS' is currently the preferred term. First, it is less medicalised and therefore fits better in non-clinical settings such as people's own homes or residential facilities, and with clients who are not ill. Second, it is less likely to be confused with other medical words

Table 14 Direct intervention techniques that target oral preparatory and oral stage difficulties

Technique	Rationale	Instructions to client	Evidence base
Oromotor exercises: Tongue exercises	Increased tongue mobility and strength improve lingual manipulation of the bolus and anterior-posterior transference of the bolus.	'Stick out your tongue. Retract your tongue.' 'Move your tongue from side to side.' 'Lick around your lips as if you are licking off sugar from a doughnut.' 'Push your tongue into your cheek while pressing on the outside of your cheek with your finger.'	Hwang et al, 2019.
Lip exercises	Greater lip mobility and strength improve lip seal (and therefore intra-oral pressure) and help with taking food off a spoon and fluid from a cup.	'Hold a tongue depressor between your lips.' 'Alternate saying "oo" and "ee."' 'Take a breath. Puff up your cheeks with air and hold.'	See Langmore and Pisegna (2015) for a critique of oromotor exercises in general.
Soft palate exercises	Increased mobility and strength of the velum improve velopharyngeal competence, which in turn aids intraoral pressure and prevents nasal regurgitation.	'Take a breath. Puff up your cheeks with air and hold.' 'Alternate /m/ and /b/.'	

(*Continued*)

Table 14 (Continued)

Technique	Rationale	Instructions to client	Evidence base
Desensitisation	Hypersensitivity to touch which causes abnormal or primitive oral reflexes (eg, bite reflex, rooting, bruxism) can be lessened by using sustained and systematic touch. Reduction in bite reflex enables better oral care and facilitates the introduction of oral food and drink.	The instructions will depend on the client. With some people who are highly sensitive, you will need to start by touching distal parts of the body, such as the hands. Gradually work your way up – using firm but gentle touch on the arms, shoulders, head and face – until the person can tolerate being touched around the mouth (ie, without a reflexive reaction being triggered). This needs to be carried out several times a day, so you can teach relatives and carers to do this.	Gilmore et al, 2003.
IOPI®	Increases lip and tongue strength, thereby improving lip seal and lingual manipulation of the bolus.	According to manufacturer.	Adams et al, 2013.
IQoro®	Increases lip and tongue strength, thereby improving lip seal and lingual manipulation of the bolus (also targets pharyngeal and oesophageal musculature).	According to manufacturer.	Hägg and Tibbling, 2016.

Table 15 Direct intervention techniques that target pharyngeal stage difficulties

Technique	Rationale	Instructions to client	Evidence base
Altering the bolus (size, texture, taste, temperature, carbonisation)	Heightening sensory awareness promotes a prompter swallow reflex.	None specific.	Roa Pauloski et al (2012). Regan (2020). Kawakami et al (2019). Sdravou, Walshe and Dagdilelis (2012).
Masako	Providing resistance to tongue movement forces the tongue base to work harder and the posterior pharyngeal wall to move more.	'Hold your tongue tip between your teeth and swallow.' This should be carried out with no food or drink in the mouth.	Fujiu and Logemann, 1996.
Shaker	Improves hyolaryngeal excursion and opening of the cricopharyngeal sphincter.	'Lie on your back and keep your head raised for one minute.' Repeat three times with a one-minute rest period between each head lift. Then carry out 30 consecutive head lifts, holding each one for two seconds. This should be carried out with no food or drink in the mouth.	Shaker et al, 1997. Mepani et al, 2009.
Chin tuck against resistance (CTAR)	Enhances suprahyoid muscle activity and therefore opening of the cricopharyngeal sphincter.	'Hold a rubber ball under your chin and push down on it.' This should be carried out with no food or drink in the mouth.	Yoon, Khoo and Rickard Liow, 2014.
CTAR-Swift			Smithard et al, 2022.

(Continued)

Table 15 (Continued)

Technique	Rationale	Instructions to client	Evidence base
Lee Silverman Voice Treatment (LSVT®)	Cricopharyngeal sphincter opens more promptly. Improves cough (and therefore airway protection).	According to LSVT® techniques (you have to be a registered LSVT® clinician with the relevant training to conduct this treatment).	Nozaki et al, 2021. Miles et al, 2017.
Expiratory Muscle Strength Training (EMST)	Improves pulmonary function by practising breathing against resistance, thereby improving airway protection and hyolaryngeal excursion.	As per device.	Troche et al, 2010. Brooks, McLaughlin and Shields, 2019.
Neuromuscular electrical stimulation (NMES)	An electrical current flows across the skin to stimulate muscular and sensory activity during a functional task, such as eating or drinking.	As per device.	Alamer, Melese and Nigussie, 2020.
Surface electromyography (sEMG)	Electrodes provide biofeedback to the client when performing a swallow or safe swallow strategy manoeuvre.	Depends on the safe swallow strategy being trialled.	Archer, Smith and Newham, 2021.
Phagenyx®	A pharyngeal electrical stimulation device which improves the neuroplasticity of the motor cortex to enhance swallow function.	None specific – a modified nasogastric tube containing electrodes is inserted into the pharynx and electrical stimulation is delivered via the electrodes for a short period of time.	See the Phagenesis website.

Table 16 Possible difficulties at each stage of the swallow

Stage	Possible swallowing difficulties
Oral preparatory	Cognitive difficulties affecting judgement, choice-making, recognition of foodstuffs and planning. Physical difficulties affecting the ability to move food/drink to the mouth. Reduced ability to open the mouth. Reduced ability to create a bolus through mastication and lingual manipulation. Reduced production of saliva (or altered consistency). Reduced ability to control the bolus. Oral residue. Pre-swallow aspiration.
Oral	Reduced ability to move the bolus from the front to the back of the mouth. Reduced control of the bolus. Reduced buccal tension. Reduced lip seal. Oral residue. Pre-swallow aspiration.
Pharyngeal	Vallecular residue. Pyriform sinus residue. Delayed swallow reflex. Velopharyngeal incompetence. Reduced epiglottic retroversion. Reduced vocal fold closure. Reduced cricopharyngeal sphincter opening. Aspiration during the swallow. Post-swallow aspiration.
Oesophageal	Reflux. Post-swallow aspiration.

beginning with the prefix 'dys-', such as dysarthria, dyspraxia and so on. This might lessen the chances of receiving confusing referrals (as I have in the past), such as 'expressive dysphagia'. There is also the acknowledgement that issues may arise with any part of the eating and drinking process, not just the physical. For example, a client with a head injury may be at risk of aspiration more because they are highly distractible at mealtimes than because of the changed physiology of their swallow. 'EDS' feels like a more inclusive term and perhaps helps us as clinicians to embrace not just the biological aspects of deglutition but also the psychosocial, spiritual and cultural factors.

> **D CLINICAL TOP TIP**
>
> In a report or in medical notes, it is good practice to categorise the dysphagia issue into severity, origin and signs – for example: 'The client presents with severe (severity) neurogenic (origin) oropharyngeal dysphagia, characterised by a swallow reflex delayed to the level of the valleculae and post-swallow aspiration on all consistencies (signs).'

E IS FOR . . .

END OF LIFE

'End-of-life care' is generally considered to be the support given to people who are expected to die within 12 months. The Health and Care Professions Council (HCPC) contributed to a document entitled *One Chance to Get it Right* (Leadership Alliance for the Care of Dying People, 2014), and SLTs have a pivotal role to play in supporting people and their EDS needs in the last year, weeks and days of life.

As people approach the last days of life, appetite may become suppressed and there may be a reduction in oral intake. People become drowsy and ultimately unresponsive; Cheyne-Stokes breathing (when respiration gets quicker, then slower and shallower until eventually it stops) may be in evidence. If you work with people entering the last weeks and days of life, you may want to familiarise yourself with these normal parts of dying, so that you can reassure relatives who may never have been in this situation before.

The SLT's role with individuals at the end of life is to maintain their comfort and dignity in relation to EDS, including promoting optimum mouthcare and management of secretions. Although the three tenets of management (safety, nutrition/hydration, quality of life) all pertain, the balance is heavily weighted towards quality of life. Deriving nutrients is not a priority at this stage; people may benefit from small tastes of a favourite flavour, such as a pudding. Food which could constitute a choking hazard should not be offered in order to avoid unnecessary distress. Keeping the person hydrated enough to be comfortable remains important and can be achieved through sips of fluid or ice chips. The dying person may experience aspiration of fluid; our job is to minimise this and maximise comfort from the fluid. We may, for example, recommend a specific head and trunk position. It is unlikely that thickened fluids will be offered at this stage, unless the client specifically requests this.

Mouthcare is central to maintaining the client's dignity and comfort. The mouth should be kept moist and clean by using non-foaming toothpastes with a soft toothbrush, lip gels (eg, Oralieve®) or a mouth hydrator.

SLT end-of-life care also includes supporting and advising loved ones. Understanding that reduced oral intake is normal at end-of-life may reassure carers and free them to offer small amounts of some favourite foods for enjoyment rather than nutrition. A build-up of secretions and overt signs of aspiration such as coughing and wet voice may be distressing for the relative; again, calm reassurance may be what is needed from the clinicians supporting them and their loved one.

ENTERAL FEEDING

Although I object to the use of the word 'feeding' in relation to giving food and drink to another adult, it feels like it is here to stay when it comes to non-oral ways of getting nutrients into the body – there just does not seem to be a better term at present.

'Enteral feeding' refers to an artificial method of nutritional intake which bypasses the mouth and pharynx (and therefore the need for swallowing). If a client is unable to derive any or enough nutrition and hydration orally, the MDT will decide on the best choice of enteral feeding for that individual, in consultation with them and/or their next-of-kin. The dietitian is the primary clinician involved in the recommendation and monitoring of enteral feeding and will advise on the safest or lowest-risk routes.

There are four main enteral feeding types:

- Nasogastric tube (NGT): A small-bore tube passed through the nose, pharynx and upper oesophageal sphincter into the oesophagus and the stomach.

- Percutaneous endoscopic gastrostomy (PEG): A tube inserted directly into the stomach.
- Radiologically inserted gastrostomy: A tube inserted with X-ray guidance.
- Percutaneous endoscopic jejunostomy (PEJ): A tube inserted directly into the small intestine.

An NGT is generally used for shorter periods of time (less than four weeks), whereas a PEG/PEJ is a more permanent option. You may also hear reference to 'parenteral feeding': this is an intravenous (ie, directly into a vein) method of getting nutrients into the body and is used if nutrients cannot be absorbed by the digestive system (eg, because of a blockage).

SLT clients may have enteral feeding because:

- they are deemed completely unsafe on any oral intake (ie, there is significant risk of aspiration) and have been made nil by mouth by the MDT;
- they are at severe risk of aspiration on oral intake and are therefore nil by mouth, but are enjoying small tastes orally for pleasure;
- they can manage some oral intake but still derive the majority of their hydration/nutrition enterally; or
- they can manage a substantial amount of food and fluid orally but need a top-up via the tube.

Some SLT clients may need enteral feeding temporarily during their rehabilitation (eg, someone who has had a stroke or is undergoing radiotherapy for head and neck cancer), while others may need enteral feeding as a permanent option (eg, those with neurodegenerative conditions or severe head injury). Either way, liaison with the dietitian is always merited to ensure that the client is maintaining optimum nutrition and hydration.

It is worth noting that sometimes enteral feeding may be contraindicated. For example, research (Finucane et al, 1999) has suggested that health and mortality are not improved by the use of enteral feeding in late-stage dementia, and that the risks outweigh any potential benefits. However, a subsequent systematic review challenged this view (Brooke and Ojo, 2015). Ethical issues abound in the late-stage dementia population which can be challenging for the clinician; the client is unlikely to have capacity to consent and quality of life can be difficult to gauge. Carers may find themselves in the invidious position of helping someone who is known to be aspirating to eat and drink. The role of the SLT here is to reassure and support the carer while ensuring that the client is eating and drinking as safely and comfortably as possible (eg, through optimum positioning).

Nutrition and hydration are, of course, basic human needs which no one can be legally deprived of. However, it has been legally argued that enteral feeding can be classed in certain circumstances as a treatment, which can be withdrawn if that is in the client's best interests. For example, in 1993, enteral feeding was deemed to be a treatment and was withdrawn in the case of Tony Bland. Tony had sustained a catastrophic anoxic brain injury during the Hillsborough disaster of 1989. EEG and CT scans showed that although his brainstem was still functioning, there was no cortical activity (and therefore no cognitive function) and no hope of recovery. Treatment was therefore deemed futile and the decision made to withdraw enteral feeding. Tony died several days after withdrawal of enteral feeding.

People with neurodegenerative conditions may draw up an advance directive which states that they do not wish to receive enteral feeding when their swallow function becomes impaired. This should be discussed with and documented by their physician.

EPIGLOTTIS/EPIGLOTTIC RETROVERSION

The epiglottis is the leaf-shaped, highly elastic cartilage which rises up from the base of the tongue. It is connected to tissues which surround it by several ligaments, whose names denote the areas of attachment:

- Hyoepiglottic ligament: Connects the epiglottis to the hyoid bone.

- Thyrohyoid ligament: Connects the hyoid bone to the thyroid cartilage.
- Thyroepiglottic ligament: Connects the epiglottis to the thyroid cartilage.

During the swallowing process, the epiglottis becomes horizontal as the hyoepiglottic ligament extends. Kitamura et al (2022) contend that there is also a tendon – which they term the 'glossoepiglottic tendon' – that originates from the posterior part of the genioglossus muscle in the tongue and attaches to the centre of the epiglottic cartilage. The supposition is that sustained contraction of the posterior part of the genioglossus muscle persistently pulls on the epiglottis, and that the relaxation of the glossoepiglottic tendon may cause the epiglottis to invert during swallowing. The bolus also has a mechanical effect on the epiglottis, causing it to invert.

The role of the epiglottis in swallowing is thus to help protect the airway (along with closure of the vocal folds and vestibular folds and forward movement of the arytenoids) in a process known as 'epiglottic retroversion'. At the point of swallow during the pharyngeal stage, the epiglottis flips down, thereby covering the entrance to the laryngeal vestibule and directing the bolus towards the oesophagus in a chute-like fashion.

The valleculae are formed by the base of the epiglottis meeting the tongue. These pockets in the pharynx can be the site of residue post-swallow and may also provide a landmark when describing a delay in the swallow reflex. For example, the clinician might state: 'The swallow is delayed to the level of the valleculae.'

Functioning of the epiglottis may be compromised through inflammation (epiglottitis) or fibrosis (stiffening) resulting from radiotherapy.

The epiglottis and its movement during the pharyngeal stage of the swallow cannot be seen during clinical examination. In order definitively to comment on the movement of the epiglottis, the clinician must carry out an instrumental assessment, such as VF or FEES.

E CLINICAL TOP TIP

Try to talk to clients with neurodegenerative conditions (eg, motor neurone disease) about the probable progression of dysphagia, the likelihood of aspiration and the possible need for enteral feeding while they still have functional speech. Some clients with progressive disorders may want to sign an advance directive stating that they do not want enteral feeding even when their swallow deteriorates to the point of aspirating on all oral intake. In this case, the SLT role becomes one of recommending consistencies and positioning which make oral intake as safe, comfortable and enjoyable as possible.

F IS FOR . . .

FIBREOPTIC ENDOSCOPIC EVALUATION OF SWALLOWING (FEES)

A CSE can tell us a lot, but sometimes we need to dig deeper – and more objectively – in order to ascertain exactly what is happening with the swallow. For example, a CSE will not tell us exactly where the bolus is at the point of swallow. It cannot tell us whether any residue is left in the pharynx post-swallow, where or how much (although skilled proponents of cervical auscultation might tell you otherwise). Likewise, a CSE cannot detect silent aspiration.

For these reasons, it may be necessary to carry out an instrumental, objective assessment after the clinical examination. These include VF, pulse oximetry and FEES. The decision to carry out an instrumental assessment may include the following considerations:

- You need to see the pharyngeal structures.
- You suspect pooling/residue in the pharynx and want to confirm and *measure this.*
- You suspect a delay in the swallow trigger and want to confirm this (*and the level to which it is delayed*).
- You want to see whether epiglottic retroversion is occurring.
- You suspect laryngeal penetration/aspiration and want to confirm this.
- You suspect silent aspiration and want to confirm this.
- *You suspect that the cricopharyngeal sphincter is not relaxing or not opening enough to allow all the food and fluid through (resulting in residue/pooling above).*

- *You suspect velopharyngeal incompetence.*
- *You want to try out some head positions or other safer swallowing strategies.*

The decision to carry out FEES rather than one of the other instrumental assessments is based on what you want to find out (the points in italics above may be better investigated using VF – see under V), but may also be influenced by the following:

- The client is unable to transfer or be transferred from bed to chair (a portable FEES might be particularly useful on the intensive care unit).
- The client has reduced cognitive and/or language abilities, making instructions difficult to follow.
- The MDT feels that exposing the client to ionising radiation (as in VF) is not appropriate.
- You want to avoid the possibility of side effects associated with VF, such as constipation from ingestion of barium.
- You want to be able to view the structures of the pharynx and larynx, including the vocal folds.

FEES must be carried out only by an SLT with specific post-registration training and experience; however, less experienced SLTs may be involved in FEES clinics under the guidance of an experienced colleague to develop their skills. The procedure involves the passing of a flexible, small-gauge tube with a camera at its end (nasendoscope) through the nose and into the pharynx in order to see the structures of the nasopharynx, oropharynx and hypopharynx. Once in situ, the nasendoscope affords a clear view of the epiglottis at rest, the base of the tongue, the pyriform sinuses, the vocal folds, the arytenoids and the trachea. You may want to assess the appearance of these structures, sensory responses, the swallow reflex and the swallowing of saliva, food and fluids.

To see the bolus clearly during FEES, clinicians often use foodstuffs which are easy to distinguish from saliva or other secretions, such as milk or custard.

One disadvantage of FEES is that it does not enable you to assess the oral preparatory or oral stages of the swallow, but you are able to see laryngeal penetration and aspiration before and after the swallow, as well as pooling and residue post-swallow. Silent aspiration can be determined by visualising overt aspiration while not hearing the client cough. Aspiration or penetration during the swallow is more difficult with FEES, as at the actual point of swallow, so-called 'white-out' occurs – the reflecting back of light from the pharyngeal tissue which obscures the picture.

FEES is relatively risk-free but can lead to epistaxis (nose-bleeds) or, very rarely, laryngospasm (when the vocal folds spasm and close, meaning that breathing is impeded).

FEES may be uncomfortable and perceived as invasive by some people, so it may not be an appropriate instrumental assessment choice for certain clients. An inability to understand what the procedure is for, how long it will take and what the results may mean might also make it undesirable for people with cognitive and/or language difficulties.

F CLINICAL TOP TIP

The point of any assessment is to guide next steps and help in your clinical decision-making. Before you refer your client to the FEES clinic, ask yourself the following questions:

- What am I unsure about following my CSE?
- Is there a hypothesis I want to test?
- Is FEES the best instrumental assessment for what I want to find out?
- How will FEES affect my clinical decision-making?
- How will FEES benefit my client?
- Will my client understand and tolerate FEES?

G IS FOR . . .

GOAL-SETTING AND MEASURING OUTCOMES

Goal-setting in EDS management helps us to focus our intervention. Ideally, goals should be client-led, functional and meaningful. Using a framework such as the International Classification of Disability, Functioning and Health (ICF) (WHO, 2001) or the biopsychosocial-spiritual model (Sulmasy, 2002) enables the clinician to look at the client in a holistic way – not just focusing on the physical, but perhaps also setting goals related to the person's environment, ability to participate in social events or religious rites, psychosocial wellbeing or quality of life. In H for holistic EDS practice, we also discuss the importance of a person's culture when considering their EDS needs.

Information-gathering (in the form of clinical and case histories), thorough assessment (clinical and possibly also instrumental), assiduous analysis of those assessments and collaborative discussions with the client and their significant others should all lead to intervention choice and the goal of that intervention. What is it that we are hoping to achieve through the intervention? How will we measure the efficacy of the intervention? How long do we expect it to take to achieve this goal?

Without goals, our intervention may be unfocussed and ineffective; we will also not know by the end of intervention whether the treatment has been successful.

It is generally recommended that goals follow the SMART acronym: specific, measurable, appropriate/achievable, realistic/relevant and timebound. However, there is some evidence to suggest that sticking rigidly to a SMART format may compromise collaborative goal-setting and render goals less client-centred

(Hersh et al, 2012). Perhaps the acronym should be adapted to C-SMART, to include the collaborative aspect.

Let's break down how to set good EDS goals, using two examples. We have a client who is currently on minimal amounts of oral intake and lacks confidence about eating – they want to be able to eat more with increased confidence.

- **Specific:** The client specifically wants to work on increasing the quantity of food that they can manage orally, as well as their confidence in doing so.
- **Measurable:** Goals have a baseline and a target, which should both be measured using the same scale. Table 17 presents two examples of baselines and targets.
  The method for measuring the goal is the same in the baseline and the target (ie, teaspoons of a specific consistency of food and a visual analogue scale respectively).
- **Achievable:** Through assessment, we have discovered that this client can manage five teaspoons of a particular consistency safely and comfortably, so the goal needs to build on what they can do. We know that they are feeling underconfident – our management is designed to raise their confidence levels.
- **Realistic:** We know that the client can manage a certain amount of this consistency safely, so we are surmising that it should be within their physical abilities to manage a small increment. Intervention also targets confidence levels, so we anticipate a small increase on the adopted scale.

Table 17 Example of EDS baselines and targets

Baseline 1	Managing five teaspoons of IDDSI Level 4 food per day.	Target 1	To manage ten teaspoons of IDDSI Level 4 food per day.
Baseline 2	Rating confidence in eating IDDSI Level 4 food at 3 on visual analogue scale (1–10).	Target 2	To rate confidence when eating IDDSI Level 4 food at 8 or higher on visual analogue scale (1–10).

- **Time-bound:** If the client is being observed while eating and their chest is being monitored regularly for any signs of aspiration, we should know within a few days whether the intervention strategies are working and the goals are met.

So, our final goals for this client might look like this:

- **Overall aim:** To eat and drink again with more confidence.
- **Goal 1:** X will be able to manage ten teaspoons of IDDSI Level 4 food with no clinical signs of aspiration by the end of the week.
- **Goal 2:** X's confidence when eating will be rated as 8 on a visual analogue scale by the end of the week.

Intervention is how we get the client from their baseline to the target. In this example, our intervention might be as set out in Table 18.

By the end of the intervention, the goal may be:

- fully met – our duty of care for that client may end or a new goal may be set;
- partially met – we may extend the time working on that same goal or alter the goal; or
- not met – we may extend the time working on that goal, alter the goal or discard the goal and plan a new, more appropriate one.

Table 18 Examples of intervention implemented to achieve goals

Intervention to achieve Goal 1	SLT to give gradually increasing amounts of IDDSI Level 4 food (yoghurt) to client each lunchtime.
	SLT to teach use of chin tuck to client to maximise airway protection.
	SLT to liaise with physio and medical staff re client's chest status.
Intervention to achieve Goal 2	SLT to have discussion with client about concerns re swallowing.
	SLT to explain how chin tuck might help protect the airway during swallowing.

The achievement of goals is one way to measure the outcome of intervention for a client; reaching the target of a goal means that your intervention has been successful. Specific outcome measurement tools are also very useful in proving the efficacy of intervention. As clinicians, we might need to show the outcome of intervention to various stakeholders, such as service commissioners, funders, managers, researchers, other members of the MDT and, of course, the client themselves.

For example, the Functional Oral Intake Scale (FOIS) (Crary, Mann and Groher, 2005) is a simple method of showing where the client was pre-treatment versus where they are post-treatment (see Table 19).

Useful as this scale is in terms of quantifying and describing oral intake as an outcome, sometimes EDS intervention is not necessarily focused on this. Our therapy goals may revolve around the client feeling more comfortable eating and drinking or participating in a family social event. Based on four of the dimensions of the ICF (WHO, 2001), Enderby and John's Therapy Outcome Measures (TOMs) (2015 and 2025) are commonly used by SLTs to determine the efficacy of functional as well as impairment-based EDS intervention. TOMs provide scales in all the main SLT diagnostic categories, including

Table 19 FOIS levels (adapted from Crary, Mann and Groher, 2005)

FOIS level	Description
FOIS Level 1	Nil by mouth – completely dependent on enteral feeding for all hydration and nutrition.
FOIS Level 2	Dependent on enteral feeding with minimal or inconsistent oral intake.
FOIS Level 3	Consistent oral intake, supplemented by enteral feeding.
FOIS Level 4	Total oral intake of one consistency only.
FOIS Level 5	Total oral intake of different consistencies requiring special preparation and/or specific compensatory strategies.
FOIS Level 6	Full oral diet with no special preparation needed but some food limitations.
FOIS Level 7	Full oral diet with no restrictions and no compensatory strategies needed.

Table 20 Goals and outcomes

Goal	OM baseline	Possible OM target
X will be able to manage ten teaspoons of IDDSI Level 4 food with no clinical signs of aspiration by the end of the week.	FOIS Level 2 TOMs (activity): 1 (oral intake insufficient to meet hydration and nutrition needs)	FOIS Level 3 TOMs (activity): 2 (additional non-oral nutrition, hydration or supplements needed)
X's confidence when eating will be rated as 8 on a visual analogue scale by the end of the week.	TOMs (wellbeing/distress): 2 (moderate consistent)	TOMs (wellbeing/distress): 4 (mild occasional)

dysphagia, which help the clinician to measure outcomes of intervention that may target body structure, activity, participation or the client's wellbeing.

If we look back at our two goals above, we could imagine the potential outcome measurements as presented in Table 20.

Setting good, clear goals is essential in order to target our intervention; and assessing the outcome of that intervention is equally important, whichever measure we use.

> **G CLINICAL TOP TIP**
>
> Setting goals and measuring outcomes are not always easy and take practice – you may gain confidence in using TOMs, for example, by pairing up with a colleague and comparing your assessment of functioning.

H IS FOR . . .

HOLISTIC EDS PRACTICE

The concept of holism in therapy relates to the ability to see the person as a whole, the sum of many parts, rather than just their illness. It challenges depersonalisation in healthcare and promotes person-centred and personalised care. I remember recovering in hospital once and being referred to as 'the ectopic in Bed 4' – a dehumanising and painful memory. Language is powerful; using shorthand is understandable in a busy working environment, but we need to be mindful of the possible effects on our patients.

Holism is closely aligned to the social model of illness and disability, in which the client is seen as the expert in their condition (Swain et al, 2013).

The three tenets of EDS management (safety, nutrition/hydration and quality of life) demand that we take a holistic view of our client and their family. That is, we need to consider all facets of their personhood: body, mind and spirit. The effects of dysphagia on an individual may be biological, psychological, social, cultural, religious or spiritual, and therefore goals and intervention may focus on any or all of these areas. During collaborative goal-setting, we need to ascertain what is meaningful to the client. One of the first questions we might ask is: what is most important to you at the moment?

This book and others on dysphagia put a lot of emphasis on the biological – what has happened to the body's structure and function. We need to know this to target our impairment-based intervention – that is, that intervention which aims to ameliorate function (eg, stimulating the swallow reflex through taste, temperature or electrical stimulation), as well as some compensation-based techniques which temporarily alter the physiology of the

DOI: 10.4324/9781003480877-8

swallow (eg, head positions). However, the client's EDS need may be impacting other domains of their life and goals might therefore be related to these.

In the 1970s, Engel first put forward the idea that psychological and social aspects as well as physical aspects of illness and disability might impact the person's life in the biopsychosocial model. In 2002, Sulmasy expanded this model to include the spiritual aspect of the client in his biopsychosocial-spiritual model. We could consider developing this model still further by adding in the cultural aspect, in a biopsychosocial-spiritual-cultural model (see Figure 1).

Why is it important to consider each of these facets of personhood in assessment of EDS needs and in our intervention? How might psychological, social, spiritual and cultural aspects affect our management?

PSYCHOLOGICAL ASPECTS

Oral intake is a basic human need and function, so it is little wonder that no longer being able to eat and drink as before (in the case of acquired dysphagia) or experiencing lifelong difficulties

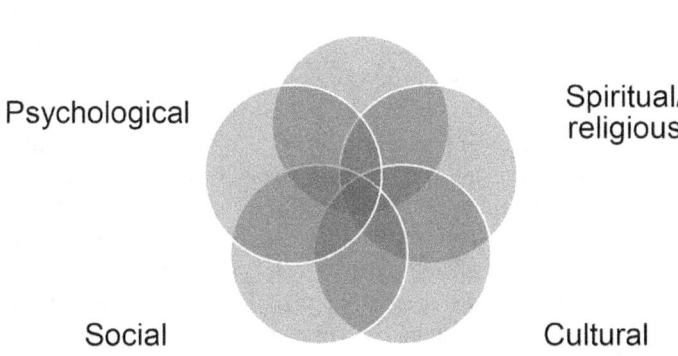

Figure 1 The interaction between biological, psychological, social, spiritual and cultural aspects of the person

with oral intake (in the case of developmental conditions) can have a profound effect on an individual's psychological health and wellbeing. People who have such severe dysphagia that they are deemed unsafe on any oral intake and therefore derive all their hydration and nutrition via other (enteral) means may experience a profound sense of loss – of enjoyment, of human interaction, of connection.

For some people, food and drink are inextricably entwined with their character, so a loss of or change in the ability to eat and drink may affect sense of self or role. Consider, for example, no longer being able to invite friends around for a meal or even a coffee, or no longer being able to meet your friends at the pub.

People who are eating and drinking orally but who experience episodes of laryngeal penetration, aspiration or even choking may feel very vulnerable and fearful. Fear may, of course, make the person reluctant to eat and drink, leading to physical consequences such as dehydration – an example of the overlapping nature of these different facets.

People with acquired conditions may already be prone to depression (eg, after stroke (Baker et al, 2020)), which may be exacerbated by the loss of enjoyment and socialisation afforded by eating and drinking.

Carers may also experience a sense of loss: loss of the companionship and enjoyment of preparing and eating food together, and socialising and celebrating with food and drink. Some carers have to take responsibility for preparing food of a particular consistency or helping their loved one to eat and drink, which can seem like a huge psychological burden. The carer of someone with an advance directive which stipulates that they want to continue to eat and drink even when their swallow deteriorates to the point of regularly aspirating may find themselves in the invidious position of helping someone to eat and drink when they know this intake is being aspirated and may cause physical harm. Even if someone is receiving sufficient nutrients via enteral means (a nasogastric tube or PEG), carers may feel that the ability to nurture and heal through food is denied them. Fear, anxiety and depression may ensue.

SOCIAL ASPECTS

Eating and drinking are about more than providing nutrients and hydration to the body. Many social events are centred around food and drink – whether happy celebrations, such as birthday parties; sad occasions, such as funerals; or work situations, such as conferences. People with EDS needs may no longer be able to eat and drink at all or may have to implement safer swallowing strategies (eg, head positions or use of adaptive cutlery) which mark them out as different and may cause embarrassment. They may experience anterior loss of saliva or food – another potential cause of embarrassment. Some clients may want to continue to be involved in these social situations, despite a limited ability to partake, but others may find this too painful and may prefer to eschew social situations.

Spouses, friends, parents and children of people with EDS needs may also find their socialisation curtailed as they opt to avoid social situations where their loved one is unable to be fully included.

SPIRITUAL/RELIGIOUS ASPECTS

Just as food and drink may be core components of social gatherings, so may they feature in many spiritual and religious practices and rites. Mathisen et al (2015) state a number of reasons for considering spirituality in SLT practice:

- Religious or spiritual beliefs can be so fundamental to an individual that ignoring these may mean that therapy becomes superficial and lack meaning.
- Good therapy outcomes may be negated by not considering spiritual issues, which may impact on the success of therapy.
- SLTs may be able to help clients access spiritual resources. In terms of EDS, this may mean safely accessing food and drink related to religious ritual, for example.

MacKenzie and Mumby (2022) argue that a person's spiritual beliefs and needs should always be integrated into therapy; to ignore this would be to ignore a fundamental aspect of that person. Let's consider four basic ways in which a person's religious and spiritual needs must be incorporated into management: ritual, fasting, feasting and requirements.

An example of ritual involving food and drink is Holy Communion taken by Christians. This comprises bread (which may be a small piece of actual bread but is more often a thin wafer made from wheat flour and water) and wine (which may be red wine or fortified wine). To most Christians, the act of taking Holy Communion (also known as the Eucharist) is a vital aspect of living out their Christianity; it symbolises the body and blood of Jesus (or his actual body and blood for Catholics) and re-enacts the Last Supper on the night before Christ's crucifixion. A Christian client with EDS needs is therefore likely to be keen to take Holy Communion, so our role might be one of seeing whether this can be done as safely as possible given their swallowing issues. For example, if their tradition involves actual bread, offering wafers which dissolve easily when mixed with saliva may be an option. Priests may also tinct – that is, dip the wafer into the wine rather than offering the cup of wine; this might be acceptable to a person for whom thin fluids are problematic. Liaison with a chaplain and discussion with the client may mean that even an individual with very significant EDS needs may still be able to tap into this important spiritual resource.

Fasting is often seen as a way of deepening one's spirituality and drawing closer to God. In Islam, for example, Muslims fast from sunrise to sunset during the month of Ramadan. This may be problematic for people who are nil by mouth because of severe dysphagia who need regular enteral feeding to maintain physical health; they may feel they are missing out on this important part of their religious observance. Referral to the chaplaincy team and/or the individual's imam for discussion may be useful here; religious leaders recognise that some rituals may not be possible for people who are unwell and can grant dispensation or just reassure the person.

Festivals in most religious traditions involve feasting. For example, the period of fasting in Ramadan mentioned above is broken by a feast known as Eid-al-Fitr where samosas, pakoras and other delicious foods are consumed. Our management for someone with EDS concerns might include discussing which foods are already of an optimum consistency or which might be modified in an acceptable and palatable way.

Certain foods may not be allowed in various religions, so we obviously need to be mindful of any prohibitions prior to commencing oral trials and when giving examples of beneficial consistencies. Table 21 presents some common prohibitions; however, not all members of a particular faith group will adhere to the same rules, so always respectfully check first.

Some world religions also have rules around preparation of food. In Judaism, for example, food must be kosher – that is, the blood must be drained from the animal or bird meat before consumption. Meat and dairy should also not be mixed together. In Islam, meat must be halal – that is, the animal must have been slaughtered according to a specific ritual.

Table 21 Religious groups and some prohibited foodstuffs

Religious group	Prohibited foodstuffs
Buddhism	Animal products (apart from yoghurt and milk). Garlic, onions and chives. Processed food.
Hinduism	Meat from any animal.
Islam	Pork. Shellfish. Alcohol.
Judaism	Pork. Shellfish.

CULTURAL ASPECTS

The *Cambridge Dictionary* defines 'culture' as 'a way of life, especially the general customs and beliefs, of a particular group of people at a particular time' (*Cambridge Dictionary*). The group might relate to the person's nationality or religious affiliation, or it might relate to their employment or societal role. The culture to which a person belongs is not always obvious to the onlooker; careful questioning and discussion will help us to gain a better understanding of a client's culture and how they identify.

At a macro level, people of the same ethnicity may say they belong to that culture. For example, a person may identify as Black British or as part of the Traveller community. However, cultural groups may also form at a more micro level, such as in a pub, an office or staffroom.

Eating and drinking may be at the heart of a culture at any level, and therefore important to an individual's sense of identity. Consider the person who goes to the pub every week to meet with their friends, drink beer and play darts. Arguably, darts at the pub is their cultural milieu. How do we integrate that person's cultural needs into our EDS management, allowing them still to engage in something that is meaningful to them and that constitutes an important part of their identity?

SUPPORTING CLIENTS' PSYCHOLOGICAL, SOCIAL, SPIRITUAL/RELIGIOUS AND CULTURAL NEEDS

Identifying the psychological, social, spiritual and cultural needs of our EDS clients is the first step, which is best done through careful case history-taking. Next, we need to ensure that we have taken these into consideration in our management. Have we set goals which incorporate these facets? In some instances, part of our management may involve referral on to someone else in the team who is better equipped to manage these aspects – for example, the clinical psychologist or chaplain. We may work collaboratively with other professionals, each bringing their own knowledge and skills to provide optimal care (see J for joint working).

MITIGATING THE POWER DIFFERENTIAL

This section began with exploring the concept of holism and aligning it with the social model of disability (Swain et al, 2013). Intrinsic to this idea is the balance of power between the clinician and the client. Holism demands that we see the client as a whole person with their own agency, and that we do not adopt a hegemonic, clinician-knows-best attitude.

In holistic practice, the clinician and client are exploring, investigating and making decisions together in an equal partnership. Practical ways to mitigate any possible power differential include the following:

- Seating and body posture: Ensure that you are at the same level as the client, possibly seated to one side and with no barriers (such as a table) between you.
- Listen as much – if not more – than you speak.
- Avoid terms such as, 'I think it would be best if . . .', 'In my experience . . .'
- Use empowering phrases such as, 'I'm interested in . . .', 'Tell me more about . . .', 'What do you think about . . .?'

As you embark on setting goals and planning intervention, ask the following questions:

- What is most important to this person at this time?
- What can I do to help?
- Have I considered all facets of their personhood (ie, physical, psychological, social, spiritual, cultural)?

NARRATIVES IN EDS NEEDS

Over the years, Frank's (2013) illness narratives (chaos, restitution and quest) have helped me to consider the illness, disability and treatment stories of clients with multifarious conditions, always keeping in mind that an 'untold story is an unheard story' (MacKenzie, 2017).

Clients' stories help us to understand their perspective, their priorities and their readiness for intervention. Listening to clients' narratives can create empathy and mitigate the possible, though perhaps sometimes unacknowledged, power differential between the clinician and the patient. As the SLT, you may be seen as the one wielding the power, with your technical knowledge and decision-making capabilities. You may be wearing a uniform that marks you out as a professional – the expert. We must ensure that we acknowledge the competence of our clients, sharing the discussion and decisions with them and giving them space and time to talk through their concerns. We will discuss this a little more under R for risk.

Although every client's story is unique to that individual, Frank (2013) asserts that there are three broad categories of illness (or disability) narrative that individuals employ when they are trying to make sense of what has happened or is happening to them. They do not necessarily occur in a linear fashion and an individual may go back and forth between them; but at the point of diagnosis, chaos is often the first and overriding story heard.

CHAOS

'Chaos' is referred to by Frank (2013) as the anti-narrative, because people deep in this narrative may be unable to articulate their distress; they are adrift, mired in physical, emotional and spiritual pain. Theirs is a hopeless story, where they see no end to the suffering and experience no hope of recovery and no one is in control or able to help. The dreadfulness of this state often cannot be put coherently into words (which, of course, is compounded in many of our clients who may also have speech, language and cognitive difficulties as well as EDS needs). Clients who are deep in chaos may be severely distressed or depressed and may not be in a place where they can even contemplate recovery. Assessment, goal-setting, therapy or recommendations may not be appropriate at this point. EDS management might simply comprise listening to the person's concerns.

RESTITUTION

Restitution fits comfortably in the medical model of illness and disability and is the antithesis of the social model. In this narrative, the patient is a passive subject of the illness (sometimes the language of passivity and victimhood is employed, such as 'suffering from', being 'confined to a wheelchair' or 'bedridden/bedbound' – and indeed, the word 'patient' itself from the Latin *'patiens'* – 'one who suffers'). The client living the restitution narrative does not take responsibility for their own recovery; the health professional is seen as the expert, called in to cure. As clinicians, we have probably all had the experience of clients and carers needing a definitive prognosis, perhaps insisting on unrealistic levels of intervention in an effort to make things better. Sometimes we may even face anger because we are seen to be not doing enough.

For EDS needs, a restitution narrative may have both a positive and negative impact on the patient. On the one hand, speaking in restitutive terms may engender hope and a desire to conquer the swallowing difficulties. Clients may adopt a lexicon of war, such as fighting the disease, not wanting to lose the battle or being brave. On the other hand, a restitution narrative may be unhelpful for clients with a degenerative condition that cannot be cured or with a permanent disability resulting from an illness. Their ability to accept changes in EDS function and to maximise enjoyment in life may be hindered by an unrealistic expectation of complete cure.

Direct therapy techniques aimed at ameliorating the swallow process might be viewed as part of the restitutive narrative; oromotor exercises and stimulation therapies promise to improve function.

QUEST

If the restitution narrative is aligned with the medical model of disability, the quest narrative is its antithesis and exemplifies the social model. In the quest narrative, people who were patient patients are now getting on with their altered lives, searching for a different way of being, with meaning and purpose. The EDS issues may not necessarily have improved or disappeared, as is longed for in the restitution narrative; but nor do they define the individual, as in the chaos narrative.

Quest-driven EDS intervention may include compensatory strategies, such as head positions. These techniques fit well into this narrative, with the therapist accompanying the individual, as together patient and therapist solve problems, set goals and compensate in order for the person with a disability or illness to live well and to experience safe, enjoyable eating and drinking again.

Understanding our client's narrative may help with clinical decision-making and goal-setting; which type of intervention aligns with their current narrative?

> **H CLINICAL TOP TIP**
>
> Live out your holistic and person-centred care ethos by using person-first language, such as 'person with EDS needs' or 'person with dysphagia' (rather than identity-first language, such as 'dysphagic person').

I IS FOR . . .

INTERNATIONAL CLASSIFICATION OF DISABILITY, FUNCTIONING AND HEALTH (ICF)

The ICF (WHO, 2001) has influenced SLT intervention-planning, goal-setting and outcome measurement for decades. As a framework, it encourages the clinician to manage the whole client, not just their impairment, so that intervention becomes client-centred and holistic. Therapy, as we know, is not necessarily about fixing the physical problem; it can be about empowering the client to adapt to and live well with a change in function.

The ICF recognises that a change to body functions and structure (which used to be termed 'impairment') can have a profound impact on a person's activity levels, which in turn can affect their ability to participate in events and pursuits which give their life meaning and purpose. Function occurs in a context, so the ICF also recognises environmental and personal factors which may impact this.

An example of mapping a client with EDS needs onto the framework is set out in Table 22.

Table 22 Mapping a client with EDS needs arising from Parkinson's disease onto the ICF health domains

ICF domain	Example of client with EDS needs
Health condition	Parkinson's disease.
Body functions and structure	Moderate oropharyngeal dysphagia.
Activity	Delay in swallow reflex with reduced airway protection – chin tuck recommended.
Participation	Reluctant to eat at social gatherings.
Environmental factors	Lack of public understanding of EDS issues.
Personal factors	Fear of coughing.

DOI: 10.4324/9781003480877-9

EDS goals and intervention may be based on any or all of the ICF domains. For example, you might set two goals with a client, one of which focuses on improving the strength of their lip seal – perhaps using a device such as the IOPI® – and one which aims to improve confidence in eating in public (perhaps by gradually introducing them to social eating situations). The first goal is very much based on body structure and function; while the second focuses more on activity and participation.

The TOMs (Enderby and John, 2015) – discussed under G for goal-setting and outcome measurement – are based on this framework, utilising the following categories to measure the efficacy of intervention: impairment, activity, participation and wellbeing.

INTERNATIONAL DYSPHAGIA DIET STANDARDISATION INITIATIVE (IDDSI)

Established in 2019, IDDSI has been adopted worldwide as a way of ensuring that the texture modification of food and fluid for safer swallowing is consistent and uniform. Prior to IDDSI, descriptive terms such as 'custard-thick' were used, with the obvious propensity for subjectivity, as well as a system of numbered and lettered stages (eg, fluid stage 2, food texture C) which – especially without reference to a key – were judged as unhelpful and open to interpretation.

There are eight IDDSI levels which comprise both fluids (from thin/normal to extremely thick – Levels 0–4) and food (from liquidised to normal – Levels 3–7). The IDDSI website contains myriad helpful resources for the clinician.

Table 23 shows examples of foods and fluids at each level. However, you must ensure that you measure each particular food type against the IDDSI standards and testing methods, and tailor the food examples to your client's preferences and culture.

IDDSI levels are also used during assessment of oral intake – see under C for clinical swallow examination.

Table 23 IDDSI levels with descriptions and examples

IDDSI level	Description	Food/fluid example
Level 0	Thin fluid.	Water, milk, squash, tea.
Level 1	Slightly thick fluid.	Fluid with thickener. Check consistency. Some drinks may be naturally slightly thick (eg, a milkshake) – always check the consistency using the IDDSI flow test.
Level 2	Mildly thick fluid.	Fluid with thickener. Check consistency. Some drinks may be naturally thick (eg, nectar) – always check consistency using the IDDSI flow test.
Level 3	Liquidised (food). Moderately thick (fluids).	Gravy. Sauces. Runny pureed fruit.
Level 4	Pureed (food). Extremely thick (fluids).	Pureed food (eg, meat). Thick cereal.
Level 5	Minced and moist.	Flaked fish in a sauce. Minced/mashed fruit and vegetables.
Level 6	Soft and bite-sized.	Stew with small soft meat and vegetable chunks. Small chunks of steamed or boiled vegetables.
Level 7	Easy to chew. Regular.	Sandwiches which can be easily broken apart with a fork. Stews with tender meat and soft vegetables.

As discussed under C for compensatory strategies, the recommendation of thickened fluids should not be considered the panacea and, as with all intervention, its efficacy and acceptability to the client must be considered carefully.

> **I CLINICAL TOP TIP**
>
> The IDDSI website includes foods that could constitute a choking hazard – that is, substances which could potentially occlude the airway if aspirated. A classic and tragic example in children (who obviously have a smaller

trachea) is whole grapes. Rather soberingly, the IDDSI examples all come from autopsy reports.

Other choking hazards include:

- nuts;
- hard, crusty bread;
- tough meat, such as steak; and
- raw vegetables and fruit.

Your recommendations for a client may include the words: 'Avoid all potential choking hazards, such as . . .'

Be circumspect when offering foods that change texture once in the mouth (eg, ice cream) and mixed consistencies (eg, cereal in milk).

J IS FOR . . .

JOINT WORKING

Although the SLT is the principal professional involved in addressing EDS needs, other members of the MDT also play key roles. Working collaboratively with other team members is always beneficial, bringing together expertise, skills and knowledge for the good of the patient. Some teams may function in a multidisciplinary way, where each discipline works individually but comes together to discuss findings and progress. Other teams are more interdisciplinary in nature and may carry out joint sessions (eg, during a kitchen activities of daily living session, an occupational therapist assesses the client's ability to make a cup of tea while you assess safe swallowing strategies as they drink the tea). Some teams may be transdisciplinary, where one discipline strays into the traditional territory of another (eg, an SLT on a home visit may ask the client about weight loss and report back to the dietitian).

In an acute setting, the MDT is often housed together in a shared office space, so that liaison is straightforward. Informal catchups are also possible on the wards. However, SLTs working out in the community may find that they have less direct access to other team members, in which case use of the telephone, Microsoft Teams or Zoom meetings and password-protected emails may be more common. Joint electronic notes help all team members to keep abreast of what is happening to the client in other contexts. If you do find that you are relatively isolated in your daily work, ensure that you instigate times to meet other team members, for both professional and social discussion.

Let's look at each potential member of the team in turn and determine the principal role that each plays in the team around the person with EDS needs. Not all teams will comprise all these professionals and there might be some specialist team members in your area of expertise that I have not included. In keeping with the book, these professionals are in alphabetical order, not order of importance!

CARER

By 'carer', I mean the family member(s) who looks after their loved one on a day-to-day basis, as well as those paid workers who may come in during the day (and night) to perform specific caring duties, such as helping the person get into bed. In either case, the caring relationship is an intimate one, with the carer being privy to many details of the client's functioning. They will probably have a good understanding of how much the client is eating and drinking, any specific difficulties they may be exhibiting, the efficacy of any implemented safer swallowing strategies, the client's general health status and so on. Helping someone to eat and drink, ensuring that the correct consistencies are provided and positioning maintained may prove stressful for some carers; our role is to provide adequate training, advice and support.

CHAPLAIN

A chaplain provides both clients and other members of the team with pastoral and spiritual support, whether they profess a religious faith or not. EDS difficulties can have profound psychological, social and spiritual effects on the individual, their loved ones and the staff who support them (see under H for holistic practice). An individual who is no longer able to eat and drink as before – perhaps they have to avoid certain consistencies or implement a head position, or maybe they are nil by mouth – may start to ask existential questions, such as 'Why is this happening to me?' and 'What's the point of life now?'

Specific religious rites and ceremonies intrinsic to an individual's spiritual life may centre around food, and working directly with the chaplain may enable the client to reconnect to something which gives meaning and purpose to their life. For example, a Christian client with dysphagia may safely be able to take Holy Communion (wafer and wine) if the SLT and chaplain work together.

CLIENT

The client is at the centre of all we do and is at the heart of the MDT. All decisions as far as possible should be collaborative and the client should be involved at all stages. Assessment, goals and interventions should all be functional and meaningful to the client.

DIETITIAN

The dietitian's role is to ensure that the client meets their nutrition and hydration requirements. If the client's ability to take food and drink orally is compromised, the dietitian will need to consider supplementing the diet in some way or providing alternative methods of getting food and drink into the body. Liaison between the dietitian and the SLT is vital, so that oral intake can be monitored and adjustments to supplementation made. For example, a client may be nil by mouth and need all hydration and nutrition via enteral or parenteral feeding. On the other hand, the SLT may be gradually reintroducing oral intake to someone who was nil by mouth with an alternative feeding method, necessitating an adjustment to enteral feeding. Other clients may have a deteriorating swallow function and be gradually moving from full oral intake to supplements to enteral feeding. A client who is managing limited amounts of oral intake may benefit from recommendation of oral supplements in the form of fortified drinks or puddings.

The dietitian monitors hydration, electrolytes, blood glucose levels, weight and body mass index (BMI), which is defined as the body mass (in kilograms) divided by the square of the height (in metres). A BMI of between 18.5 and 24.9 is considered healthy.

DOCTOR

The doctor often, but not always, heads up the MDT. In hospitals, doctors may be junior (from newly qualified to specialist registrar) or consultant. An SLT working with people with EDS needs will come across doctors from different specialisms depending on the cause of the dysphagia, such neurology, care of the elderly and ear, nose and throat (ENT). The medical status of the client is important for us to know in terms of clinical decision-making – for example, are there any indicators of infection? What is their level of arousal and their chest status?

In the community, the GP may refer a client to us if there are concerns about their swallow. We will need to report back to the GP with our findings; if thickened fluids are recommended, the GP will have to prescribe thickener.

Referral to a medic may be part of our management – for example, a client may attend the SLT outpatient clinic with concerns about their EDS. If a neurological cause is suspected (eg, the dysphagia could be indicative of the early stages of motor neurone disease), we would refer on to a neurologist for diagnosis.

HEALTHCARE ASSISTANT

The healthcare assistant may often be the person preparing a client's drinks and helping them to eat. General training in dysphagia, thickening drinks (if necessary) and how best to help someone to eat and drink can be provided by the SLT, as well as informal, bespoke training for the care of a specific client. Healthcare assistants may have detailed and useful knowledge about the client's day-to-day functioning, so it is well worth liaising with them; they may have information about how much the client has managed to eat and drink, how well the strategies are working and so on. Some settings may provide a rolling programme of dysphagia training for healthcare assistants.

NURSE

A nurse on a ward will have responsibility for a number of patients and a comprehensive understanding of all aspects of their care and their health. Nursing notes will document any changes in health status, wellbeing and functioning, including what the patient has managed to eat and drink during that shift. Qualified nurses may be trained by the SLT to screen the swallow.

Safe swallowing strategies for a specific client should be given to the nurse, who can then disseminate them to colleagues such as the nightshift nursing team and healthcare assistants.

Depending on your setting, you may come across highly specialist nurses, such as Admiral nurses (for people with dementia), Macmillan nurses (for people with cancer) and ENT nurses.

OCCUPATIONAL THERAPIST

Occupational therapists assess a person's occupation (ie, what they have to do in life) in relation to challenges experienced by illness or disability. Barriers to safe eating and drinking may be overcome or lessened by the use of adaptive cutlery and crockery – for example, a client who eats very slowly may need a heated plate in order still to derive enjoyment from a meal (and hopefully to finish it). The oral preparatory phase of the swallow may be enhanced by using adaptive cutlery which enables the person to continue to eat by themselves, rather than relying on someone else to help them. Occupational therapists are also experts in positioning the client and ensuring that seating systems are providing optimal support; they may recommend an addition to a wheelchair such as a headrest or tray which facilitates optimal positioning for eating and drinking. A client will be able to concentrate more on their swallow if they are not constantly concerned with trying to maintain their own sitting balance.

Occupational therapists and SLTs may well work together to achieve client goals – for example, the SLT could take part in an occupational therapist kitchen assessment, where the occupational therapist works on the client's ability to prepare food and the SLT assesses their ability safely to eat the meal.

PHARMACIST

Close liaison with the pharmacist is important for a number of reasons. Medications may have a detrimental effect on the swallow process, such as reducing or increasing saliva production (see under M for medication for some examples). Conversely, medication may temporarily improve function (eg, the use of Levodopa in patients with Parkinson's disease).

Adults with EDS needs may have to take several different drugs orally, some of which may be problematic with an impaired swallow. If someone has reduced oral control or a delayed swallow trigger, for example, a large tablet might constitute a choking hazard and an alternative formulation will need to be negotiated with the pharmacist.

PHYSIOTHERAPIST

Physiotherapists play an important role in promoting and optimising movement and function during recovery from illness or injury. They use patient-centred exercise programmes, manual therapy and rehabilitation techniques to optimise mobility and improve physical wellbeing. In particular, a physiotherapist will support patients with long-term and degenerative conditions through assessment and management of their musculoskeletal, neurological and cardiorespiratory systems. Clients with EDS needs may have or be at risk of a compromised respiratory system, so mobilisation by a physiotherapist is key.

Sometimes a client may be referred for a swallow assessment who is in a poor position for safe swallowing; they may be supine in a non-profiling bed or slumped to one side in a chair. Our physiotherapist and occupational therapist colleagues both have expertise in repositioning people, and we may need to call on their skills before we continue with the swallow assessment.

PHYSIOTHERAPIST (RESPIRATORY)

Respiratory physiotherapists have in-depth knowledge of the respiratory system: they are able to listen to breath sounds in the lungs (auscultation), interpret chest X-rays and manage respiratory secretions through a variety of invasive and non-invasive techniques, such as suction, cough assist and breathing and drainage techniques – all of which are important in

EDS assessment and management. For example, in a joint session, the respiratory physiotherapist will be able to auscultate the lungs before, during and after oral trials delivered by the SLT, thereby supporting assessment alongside the medical team if aspiration has taken place. Their skill at reading chest X-rays will help to determine whether there is consolidation of aspirate in the lungs. Their skills in airway clearance will help to support the SLT by optimising respiratory function and reducing the work of breathing prior to EDS assessment. If a client has aspirated, the respiratory physiotherapist can implement strategies to try to clear the lungs. The respiratory physiotherapist should always be summoned if a client aspirates during VF.

PSYCHOLOGIST

Clinical psychologists (and counsellors) may have a key role to play in helping a person with EDS needs come to terms with their diagnosis and changed ability to eat and drink. Clients with functional dysphagia may find a psychological approach (eg, cognitive behavioural therapy) particularly helpful, along with symptom-based techniques from an SLT.

RADIOLOGIST

A radiologist is a medical doctor who specialises in X-rays. They may be present in the VF clinic, although these days it is more common for the VF clinic to be run by the SLT and radiographer, with recourse to the radiologist for specific advice if and when necessary.

RADIOGRAPHER

Diagnostic and therapeutic radiographers are registered HCPC allied health professionals.

In EDS assessment and management, we most commonly work with diagnostic radiographers in the VF clinic. They have an excellent understanding of safety in the clinic and will ensure that all staff members are protected and that the client is not overexposed to ionising radiation. They operate the imaging equipment, reassure the client and ensure that optimal images are achieved. Diagnostic radiographers will also be responsible for undertaking CT and MRI examinations to image head and neck cancers.

Therapeutic radiographers are involved in planning and delivering the radiotherapy treatment for head and neck cancer clients and managing side effects. They will accompany clients through their radiotherapy treatment for head and neck cancer, supporting and advising patients as they progress through their treatment period. Treatment is often delivered on a daily basis for a number of weeks, so therapeutic radiographers become a familiar face.

SLTs, dietitians, doctors, physiotherapists and occupational therapists will often time their regular consultations to coincide with these daily visits, so that clients are not expected to attend hospital more frequently or for any longer than is necessary at what is a physically and emotionally exhausting time for them. Head and neck cancer MDTs, which include the therapeutic radiographer and SLT, often meet regularly as a large team to discuss every aspect of the client's treatment to ensure connected, personalised care.

SPEECH AND LANGUAGE THERAPY ASSISTANT

With good training and support, a Band 3 or 4 speech and language therapy assistant can carry out a multitude of EDS-related tasks. They may be able to help with triage of clients by taking a clinical history from medical notes and assisting the SLT to prioritise patients in order of need. The speech and language therapy assistant can be trained to carry out mealtime observations and report back any concerns to the SLT, carry out therapy packages (eg, stimulation techniques or oromotor exercises), create signage to display recommendations and check that these are being adhered to.

SPEECH AND LANGUAGE THERAPY STUDENT

Speech and language therapy students will play an active role in dysphagia assessment and management while on placement, and are therefore important members of the EDS team. Early on during their course, they may take a clinical history from the medical notes, as well as a case history from the client or family member, and carry out intervention planned by their practice educator. As they progress through their placements and become more skilled and knowledgeable, they will be able to carry out clinical assessments, analyse the results, set goals, have discussions with clients, carers and MDT members and plan intervention, in consultation with the supervising SLT.

Although speech and language therapy students are expected to know about more advanced EDS issues, such as tracheostomy and VF (and they will learn some theory at university), post-registration training and experience will be necessary for them to work autonomously in these areas. However, speech and language therapy students may participate in more complex dysphagia assessment and management under the close guidance of a qualified SLT. For example, a student SLT might help to mix the contrast material in with the foodstuffs during a VF, or they might attach a speaking valve to the client's tracheostomy tube.

J CLINICAL TOP TIP

In-service training sessions are a great way to share knowledge and skills with the rest of the MDT. Why not plan a training session where you talk about roles, responsibilities and remits of different team members? Not everyone in the team may know that SLTs are the experts when it comes to EDS and, conversely, we might not have a full understanding of what other team members can offer.

K IS FOR . . .

KEEP REFLECTING AND LEARNING

REFLECTION

Reflective practice is not only an SLT professional imperative but also an invaluable way to develop and grow as a clinician.

Intrinsic to reflection is contemplating what we have learned and what we would do differently if faced with a similar scenario in the future. One trap that we all fall into is describing the event in detail but forgetting to analyse how we felt, what we could have done differently and what our next steps are. Another pitfall to avoid is describing what the client did and did not do, instead of focusing on our own performance as a clinician. As you begin your career, you may find the use of established reflection frameworks helpful. These frameworks offer a structure of what happened, what this means and how this will alter your practice going forward. You might want to explore various published frameworks as you reflect on your EDS development, to discover which suits you best. My own suggested reflection framework is set out in Table 24.

We need to write formal reflections regularly throughout our careers – not least because our regulatory and professional bodies expect this of us. However, reflection may also be informal and verbal, taking the form of discussing cases and clients in supervision with a colleague or practice educator or presenting cases during a peer learning session.

CONTINUING PROFESSIONAL DEVELOPMENT (CPD)

Dysphagia is constantly evolving as a clinical area with new assessments and interventions emerging all the time; as in all

Table 24 EDS reflection template

EDS reflection template	
What kind of session was it (eg, assessment, intervention, advice-giving)?	
Who was involved in the session?	
What happened?	
What went well? Why was this?	
What did not go well? Why was this?	
Would you change any clinical decisions?	
Would you change any behaviours?	
Would you change any resources?	
What have you learned?	

SLT clinical areas, we must keep up to date with changes and innovations through assiduous and regular continuing professional development (CPD). Annual appraisals are a good mechanism for identifying training and development needs.

CPD opportunities may comprise formal training and educational courses (including master's level dysphagia-specific modules). However, if expense and time constraints preclude these opportunities, you can still develop your skills through:

- reading journal articles and summarising findings for your SLT team or MDT;
- shadowing more experienced colleagues or those working in a different clinical area;
- encouraging your team to invest in new EDS publications; and
- following experienced clinicians and educators on social media.

KILLIAN'S TRIANGLE

Situated in the pharyngeal wall just above the cricopharyngeus muscle is an area known as 'Killian's triangle' (sometimes referred to as 'Killian's dehiscence'), formed by two parts of the inferior pharyngeal constrictors and the cricopharyngeus. This constitutes a weak spot in the pharynx, where a pharyngeal pouch (sometimes referred to as a Zenker's diverticulum) is most likely to form. Symptoms of a pharyngeal pouch to look out for clinically include discomfort, halitosis and regurgitation. Bolus residue in the pouch can be seen on VF, and with this residue comes the risk of aspiration post-swallow when the airway is open and unprotected.

> **K CLINICAL TOP TIP**
>
> As a student, buy a notebook to record all your EDS hours, experiences and reflections. This will enable you to discuss your progress with your practice educator, plan EDS learning objectives and record evidence for competency sign-off. Once you are qualified and have met your EDS competencies, the learning continues as you begin the journey to autonomy; think about keeping a handwritten reflective log, where you can jot down reflections on a regular basis. I always find writing by hand deepens my thinking!

L IS FOR . . .

LARYNX

The pharynx leads into the larynx anteriorly and the oesophagus posteriorly. With the respiratory and digestive systems being so anatomically close, the larynx needs to be able to protect the airway from food and fluid entering during the EDS process. It does this in a number of different ways:

- closure of the true vocal folds;
- approximation of the false vocal folds (vestibular folds); and
- abrupt abduction of the vocal folds (in the form of a cough) which helps to expel foreign bodies which may inadvertently penetrate the larynx

LARYNGEAL ANATOMY, PHYSIOLOGY, FUNCTION AND INNERVATION

Let's now consider the anatomy, neuroanatomy and physiology of the larynx, as well as how we might assess the function of the larynx (and therefore the efficacy of airway protection) during the swallow evaluation.

The larynx sits at the top of the trachea and comprises the glottis (ie, the true and false vocal (vestibular) folds), the supraglottic region (from the inferior boundary of the hyoid bone to the vestibular and vocal folds) and the subglottic region (below the level of the vocal folds). The area between the vestibular folds and the entrance to the laryngeal inlet (ie, the base of the epiglottis) is sometimes referred to as the 'laryngeal vestibule'.

DOI: 10.4324/9781003480877-12

The larynx comprises several cartilages:

- the epiglottis (this also has a significant role in protecting the airway – see E for epiglottis);
- thyroid (shield-shaped) cartilage which surrounds and protects the vocal folds. The two sides (lamina) of the thyroid cartilage join to form the laryngeal prominence, which is generally more noticeable in cis men than cis women, because of the relative difference in length of the vocal folds housed within;
- cricoid (ring-shaped) cartilage, which sits below the thyroid cartilage;
- arytenoid cartilages, which move to open and close the vocal folds; and
- corniculate cartilages, which support the vocal folds.

There are no bones in the larynx. The top of the larynx is boundaried by the hyoid bone (from the Greek '*huoeidēs*', meaning shaped like the letter upsilon (υ)), which carries the distinction of being the only bone in the human body not to have articulation with another bone. The hyoid is attached to the tongue by the hyoglossus muscle (muscles are often named for their places of origin and insertion – in this case, the hyoid and glossus (tongue)). The suprahyoid muscles link the hyoid to the mandible and comprise the digastric, stylohyoid and mylohyoid muscles. The infrahyoid muscles link the hyoid to the larynx and comprise the omohyoid, thyrohyoid, sternohyoid and sternothyroid muscles.

There are also intrinsic laryngeal muscles: the posterior cricoarytenoid muscles abduct (open) the vocal folds; the lateral cricoarytenoid and interarytenoid muscles adduct (close) the vocal folds; and the cricothyroid and thyroarytenoid muscles alter the length, tension and thickness of the vocal folds.

The larynx is innervated by CN X (the vagus), which originates from the medulla in the brainstem. Superior laryngeal nerves branch off to form the internal and external laryngeal nerves. The internal laryngeal nerves supply the mucosa of the laryngeal vestibule, so are important in the initiation of a protective cough. The external laryngeal nerves supply the cricothyroid muscles, which are responsible for altering the length of the vocal folds. The right and left recurrent laryngeal nerves branch off from the vagus down in the thorax (the vagus is a long, meandering nerve – hence its name which derives from the Latin for 'wandering'). The recurrent laryngeal nerves innervate all the intrinsic muscles of the larynx except the cricothyroid muscles; most pairs of intrinsic muscles are innervated by the ipsilateral branch of the recurrent laryngeal nerve. The recurrent laryngeal nerves carry approximately 30% of the sensory information from the larynx, the superior laryngeal nerves playing a larger role in the cough reflex. Any damage to CN X – whether neurological or surgical – can have a profound effect on a person's ability to protect their airway during swallowing.

LARYNGEAL OR HYOLARYNGEAL EXCURSION

During the pharyngeal stage of the swallow process, the hyoid bone and larynx both rise upwards and forwards by contraction of the suprahyoid muscles in a motion known as hyolaryngeal excursion. This excursion effectively moves the larynx away from the pathway of the bolus, narrows the laryngeal vestibule, dilates the oropharynx and contributes to the opening of the cricopharyngeal (upper oesophageal) sphincter, which allows the bolus to enter the oesophagus.

If hyolaryngeal excursion is reduced, the airway is less protected from food or fluid, with the resultant possibility of laryngeal penetration, aspiration or choking. Impaired hyolaryngeal excursion may also result in reduced cricopharyngeal opening, thereby creating potential residue above the sphincter, with subsequent overspill of that residue into the unprotected laryngeal vestibule.

Aetiologies in which reduced hyolaryngeal excursion may be a factor include brainstem stroke and Parkinson's disease.

LARYNGEAL PALPATION

Because of the importance of hyolaryngeal excursion in the safety of the swallow, SLTs often feel this movement as part of their clinical evaluation, in a process known as laryngeal palpation. First propounded by Logemann (1996), movement of the larynx during a swallow is felt by placing the fingers thus:

- forefinger under the chin just behind the bony mandible;
- middle finger on the hyoid bone;
- ring finger on the thyroid cartilage; and
- little finger below the thyroid cartilage.

Table 25 should help you memorise the finger positioning:

Table 25 Simplified finger placement for laryngeal palpation

Fore	Fleshy bit
Middle	Hyoid
Ring	Thyroid
Little	Just below

The SLT asks the patient to swallow their saliva (known as a dry swallow) while they feel the movement of the larynx. The technique may also be used with clients who are swallowing food or drink; however, it is worth considering that the very presence of the clinician's hand makes the process less natural and therefore the findings may not be representative of the usual swallow.

Palpation allows the clinician to feel the tongue movement (including lack of movement, strength and any repetitive tongue-pumping) with their forefinger, as well as the extent and strength of hyoid and laryngeal excursion. You may also be able to estimate the oral and pharyngeal transit times, based on the movements of the structures.

It is often easier to carry out accurate laryngeal palpation on a cis male because the laryngeal prominence is more obvious and easier to feel. However, asking the client to voice may enable you to find the level of the vocal folds by feeling the vibration.

Positioning (eg, someone with kyphosis), excess submental tissue and cognitive or language issues affecting the client's understanding of the procedure may all preclude the use of laryngeal palpation with some clients.

Laryngeal cancer may necessitate the partial or complete removal of the larynx. Total laryngectomy results in the remaining trachea and the oesophagus no longer sharing a common structure in the form of the pharynx. With the respiratory and digestive systems now being completely separate, there is ostensibly no possibility of aspiration. However, during the laryngectomy procedure, the surgeon makes a small hole or fistula in preparation for the voice restoration valve, which means that aspiration becomes possible again (see A for aetiologies (structural)).

Laryngeal palpation is obviously not an option for a laryngectomy but it may still be possible and desirable to feel hyolaryngeal excursion on a client with a tracheostomy tube in situ. Evidence is equivocal regarding the effect of the presence of a tracheostomy on laryngeal movement during the swallow (Amathieu et al 2012; Kang et al, 2012), and you may also need to alter finger positioning to accommodate the tracheostomy tube.

Although laryngeal palpation has been an established element of the CSE for several decades, recent literature has suggested that, while perceptual methods such as this may *contribute* to clinical decision-making, clinicians should remain circumspect when making definitive judgements about hyolaryngeal excursion – and therefore about airway protection and cricopharyngeal opening – based solely on this method (Brates, Molfenter and Thibeault, 2019).

HYOLARYNGEAL EXCURSION AND TREATMENT OPTIONS

Some treatment techniques are predicated on this hyolaryngeal movement and its role in airway protection. For example, in the Mendelsohn manoeuvre, the client is made aware of the elevation of the larynx and is encouraged to hold the larynx in this elevated position before completing the swallow. In the chin tuck safer swallowing position, the range of laryngeal excursion is restricted and the entrance to the airway narrowed. The Shaker exercise aims to increase anterior hyolaryngeal excursion and cricopharyngeal sphincter opening by strengthening the suprahyoid muscles and enhancing thyrohyoid shortening. See under C for compensatory strategies for more details of these and other techniques.

COUGH AND COUGH TESTING

As soon as material enters the laryngeal vestibule and makes contact with the laryngeal mucosa, a cough reflex is triggered which effectively ejects the material back out into the pharynx and away from the airway. The cough involves deep inspiration, accompanied by contraction of the abdominal muscles to increase pressure in the thorax and sharp abduction of the vocal folds.

As we have seen, the afferent pathway for the cough reflex comprises sensory nerve fibres of the vagus (CN X) which travel from irritant receptors in the laryngeal mucosa to the medulla in the brainstem. A cough centre is located in the pons in the brainstem and efferent impulses from the pons then travel down the vagal (laryngeal branches), phrenic and spinal motor nerves.

The cough is a protective reflex; if an individual has a normal and robust cough reflex, often just allowing them time and reassurance will be intervention enough and there should be no further repercussions. However, coughing while eating and drinking may also be one of the signs of habitual laryngeal penetration, which may indicate a disrupted swallow and the risk of aspiration.

Clients with neurological impairment may present with a weakened cough reflex because of damage to CN X; these individuals are at risk of aspiration because of a reduced ability to protect the airway. If the cough is compromised and therefore not effective at protecting the airway, other methods of doing so need to be considered in management (eg, a head position such as a chin tuck, a swallow exercise such as the Shaker or a manoeuvre such as the supraglottic swallow – see C for compensatory therapy techniques).

Older clients may present with sarcopenia: a general weakness of muscles, including those of the larynx and of respiration (diaphragm and intercostals). Sarcopenic individuals may therefore present with a compromised swallow and reduced airway protection.

As part of your clinical EDS assessment, you may want to ascertain the strength and efficacy of the cough. This might simply take the form of asking the client to cough and assessing the perceptual strength. It is worth mentioning that this volitional cough involves a slightly different neurological process from a spontaneous (reflexive) cough, as it is mediated by the cortex. You may want to set up a cough diary, where carers and other team members record the client's coughs in terms of frequency, strength and precursor.

To assess the cough reflex itself, a tussive (cough-inducing) substance may be introduced to the client and the resultant cough assessed for strength and therefore efficacy.

> **L CLINICAL TOP TIP**
>
> When carrying out laryngeal palpation, stand to the right of your seated client (if you are right-handed – reverse this if you are left-handed) and place your left hand gently on the top of the patient's head to stop them from lifting the chin – patients often do this subconsciously in an effort to help the clinician but in fact this alters normal swallow physiology. Remember the optimal finger positioning, recognising that this is not always possible with all clients:
>
> | Fore | Fleshy bit |
> |---|---|
> | Middle | Hyoid |
> | Ring | Thyroid |
> | Little | Just below |
>
> When giving instructions to the client, use the phrase, 'I'm going to place my fingers under your chin', rather than '. . . on your throat/neck'. Reference to the neck or

throat can sound slightly threatening, making clients tense up a little. This subtle change in vocabulary can make a significant difference.

If you need to feel a second swallow, make sure that you give the client plenty of time between each, as it is difficult to effect an immediate second swallow – perhaps use some seconds to discuss their experience of the swallow difficulty.

M IS FOR . . .

MASTICATION

'Mastication' means chewing and involves the lateral movement of the jaw to move the bottom teeth in the mandible against the top teeth in the maxilla, thereby breaking down food into a cohesive mass or bolus (along with the addition of saliva and movement of the tongue). Mastication is therefore an important part of the oral preparatory stage of swallowing. The muscles of mastication include the temporalis, masseter and pterygoids, which are all innervated by CN V (trigeminal). These muscles may be assessed during a CNA by asking the client to move their jaw from side to side. Clients with damage to CN V (perhaps because of a brain injury or neurodegenerative condition) may have impaired ability to masticate; intervention may include providing consistencies which require less chewing (eg, IDDSI Level 4 or 5). Lack of dentition will, of course, also affect the efficacy of mastication.

MEDICATION

An awareness of the client's medication regimen is important for the EDS clinician for three main reasons. First, the client's swallow status may mean that certain preparations of medication are more difficult or less safe to swallow. For example, someone with a delayed swallow reflex should not be offered a solid tablet or capsule, as this could constitute a choking hazard; the tablet may enter the pharynx before the swallow reflex is triggered and therefore before the airway is shut off by the epiglottis, vestibular folds and vocal folds. It may be possible for the pharmacist to prescribe the same or similar medication in a different form – for example, as a suppository, injection or patch.

DOI: 10.4324/9781003480877-13

Table 26 Common medications and their EDS-related side effects

Medication	Used to treat	Side effect	Effect on swallowing
SSRIs	Depression	Xerostomia	Bolus formation
Antihistamine	Allergies (eg, hay fever)	Xerostomia	Bolus formation
Clozapine	Psychosis	Sialorrhoea	Saliva escape (anterior out of mouth and posterior into pharynx)
Baclofen	Muscle hypertonicity	Reduced voluntary muscle movement	Reduced ability to manipulate and control the bolus, reduced pharyngeal constriction

Second, some medications may affect the swallow process, even in people who have no pre-existing dysphagia. Table 26 shows some common medications and their EDS-related possible side effects.

Third, some medication to manage a condition may temporarily improve the swallow (eg, Levodopa for Parkinson's disease). Clients may need to be reminded to eat and drink when the positive effects of the medication are at their height. You also need to keep these on-off effects in mind when planning your assessment and reviews.

Checking the medical notes for drug history and asking the client about what medication they currently take as part of the case history are important aspects of the information-gathering process and liaison with the pharmacist can be very useful.

> **M CLINICAL TOP TIP**
>
> Make a note of current medication that your client is on – look up their common side effects or ask the pharmacist in your team. If you are struggling to understand why your client is having a particular difficulty with their EDS, it is always worth considering the effects of medication or combinations of drugs.

N IS FOR . . .

NIL BY MOUTH (NBM)/*NIL PER OS* (NPO)

The job of the SLT is to assess EDS and make recommendations for management. If the swallow is significantly impaired and the individual is deemed to be at severe risk of aspirating material, the team may decide to make the individual nil by mouth (or sometimes *nil per os* in the United States). This is not an SLT decision; rather, we contribute to the team decision by giving our opinion on the swallow function. In our notes, we might state that the client is at severe risk of aspiration on all consistencies. A nil by mouth decision is a serious one which can have a profound effect on quality of life for the individual and their significant others. Regular reviews for any change in function are merited, so that clients are not left nil by mouth for longer than is absolutely necessary. For clients who do have to remain nil by mouth for any length of time (sometimes forever), trials of safe tastes for pleasure should be considered (see under T for tastes for pleasure).

NEUROLOGICAL UNDERPINNINGS

Both the central nervous system (comprising the cortex and some subcortical structures) and the peripheral nervous system (comprising the cranial nerves and the autonomic nervous system) are involved in the swallow process. Both the efferent (motor) and afferent (sensory) pathways are important. Afferent messages are received in the nucleus tractus solitarius – sensory input is received from the tongue, lips, pharynx etc by the trigeminal, facial, glossopharyngeal or vagal nerves. Efferent messages are sent from the nucleus ambiguus to the relevant muscle end plates. The nucleus ambiguus comprises the motor nuclei of CNs V (trigeminal), VII (facial), X (vagus) and XII (hypoglossal). The autonomic nervous system regulates saliva production and peristalsis.

The volitional stages of the swallow – the oral preparatory and oral stages – are governed by the pre-frontal cortex and parts of the cortex (eg, the sensory and motor cortices). Upper motor and sensory neurones travel to and from these cortices, synapsing in the brainstem with the cranial nerves. The reflexive pharyngeal stage is governed by an area of the sensorimotor cortex in the parietal lobe.

THE CRANIAL NERVES

Six of the 12 pairs of cranial nerves are directly involved in the swallow process (as well as CN I (olfactory) for smelling food and CN II (optic) for seeing food), as outlined in Table 27.

Bilateral and unilateral innervation is clinically relevant for the SLT.

All the cranial nerves are paired, with either bilateral or unilateral (contralateral) innervation – that is, they receive messages from either both sides of the cortex (bilateral) or one side only (unilateral). 'Contralateral' refers to the fact that these upper motor neurones synapse with cranial nerves on the opposite side of the body.

Let's look at a clinical example to illustrate the difference between bilateral and unilateral innervation. If a client has a stroke which affects their right motor cortex, movement of the jaw will not be affected. This is because although the right upper motor neurone has been destroyed, the left upper motor neurone is still intact and can still synapse with the nuclei of CN V in the pons. However, the same client might well have a left-sided facial (lower face) weakness because the left lower branch of CN VII is innervated only by upper motor neurones from the right motor cortex – there is no other route to compensate. This same client may also have a weakness to the left side of the tongue (and subsequent deviation of the tongue to the left on protrusion) because CN XII is also unilaterally

Table 27 Cranial nerves involved in EDS, their origin, bilateral or unilateral innervation and motor and sensory functions

Cranial nerve (number)	Cranial nerve (name)	Originates from	Unilateral/bilateral innervation	Motor function	Sensory function
V	Trigeminal	Pons	Bilateral	Jaw movement (muscles of mastication).	Lips, oral mucosa and gingiva (gums).
VII	Facial	Pons	Top two branches: bilateral. Lower branch: unilateral.	Lip movement and closure. Buccal tension	Taste to anterior two-thirds of the tongue. Salivary glands (sublingual, submandibular).
IX	Glossopharyngeal	Medulla	Bilateral	Elevation of the larynx and pharynx. Dilation of the pharynx (stylopharyngeus muscle).	Taste to posterior one-third of the tongue.
X	Vagus	Medulla	Bilateral	Tongue base retraction (palatoglossus). Constriction of the pharynx. Elevation of the velum. Closure of the vocal folds. Reflexive, volitional and evoked cough.	Larynx and pharynx.
XI	Accessory	Medulla (and upper cervical spinal cord)	Bilateral	Head and shoulder movements. Tilt and rotation of head.	None.
XII	Hypoglossal	Medulla	Unilateral	Movement of all intrinsic and most extrinsic muscles of the tongue (except the palatoglossus).	None.

innervated; if the UMNs originating from the right motor cortex are damaged, only the left UMNs (supplying the right side of the tongue) will work.

Just a couple of caveats while we are talking about bilateral innervation. In the first few hours post neurological insult, it is not unusual to see some unilateral weakness of areas that are bilaterally innervated (eg, the upper face). This is because it sometimes takes a few hours for the other side to take over the role. In addition, bilateral innervation may be asymmetrical, so that one side is more dominant than the other (often the left). This goes some way to explain, for example, pharyngeal weakness post-unilateral stroke.

Clinical assessment of the swallow often begins with evaluating the movements and sensation of the structures involved using the order of the cranial nerves to provide a logical structure (see C for cranial nerve assessment).

> **N CLINICAL TOP TIP**
>
> The 12 cranial nerves are: olfactory, optic, oculomotor, trochlear, trigeminal, abducens, facial, vestibulocochlear, glossopharyngeal, vagus, accessory, hypoglossal (O, O, O, T, T, A, F, V, G, V, A, H).
>
> Try to memorise the cranial nerves. You might want to create your own mnemonic to help you remember them in order. There are also plenty online (some are ruder than others!) or you can use this one:
>
> > Old Onions Ordinarily Taste Terrible, Although For Vegetarian Gastronomes, Vinegar Adds Hope
>
> and here's one for the EDS-specific CNs:
>
> > Tigers Find Gorillas Very Humorous

O IS FOR . . .

ODYNOPHAGIA

Pain experienced when swallowing is known as 'odynophagia' and may occur in clients undergoing radiotherapy for head and neck cancer, those with osteophytes and in functional conditions.

Odynophagia caused by radiotherapy-induced mucositis is usually temporary; the soreness should subside as the effects of the radiotherapy wear off (a few weeks after the cessation of treatment). While the client is experiencing pain on swallowing, measures such as recommending softer consistencies may be beneficial. Sometimes odynophagia is so acute during radiotherapy that the client is unable to tolerate any oral intake and may temporarily derive all their nutrition and hydration via a PEG (see E for enteral feeding). Gradual reintroduction of oral intake can be overseen by the SLT as the mucositis resolves.

Pain from osteophytes may be managed by texture modification or ultimately surgery (see under P for presbyphagia).

Odynophagia experienced by a client with a functional disorder may be addressed via psychological and symptomatic management (read more about treatment principles for functional swallowing issues under A for aetiologies).

ORAL HYGIENE, ORAL EXAMINATION AND ORAL CARE

Good oral hygiene is important for reasons of dignity, comfort and health. Poor oral hygiene may result in the presence of oral bacteria, oral thrush and halitosis.

Clients with EDS needs may present with oral hygiene challenges for the following reasons:

- They are too unwell to carry out their own effective oral care;
- Their arousal level is low, leading to mouth breathing;
- They swallow less frequently (production and swallowing of saliva have a cleansing effect); or
- There is food residue in the oral cavity after eating.

Aspiration pneumonia is more likely to occur if the aspirate contains harmful bacteria, so oral care is of paramount importance for people with a compromised swallow. There is also evidence to suggest that poor oral hygiene and periodontal disease are associated with atherosclerotic vascular and cardiovascular disease (Dietrich et al, 2017), because bacteria from infected gums can travel around the body and cause inflammation of blood vessels and heart valves.

Examination for oral hygiene forms part of the general oromotor examination. With the client holding their mouth open, and using a pen torch to enable good visualisation of the inside of the oral cavity, the clinician looks for the concerns outlined in Table 28.

Table 28 Oral hygiene concerns, what these might indicate and possible next steps.

Oral hygiene concern	What this might indicate	Possible next steps
Dry, cracked lips and tongue	Dehydration/lack of fluid intake. Habitual mouth-breathing.	Liaise with MDT about fluid intake.
White patches on the tongue	Candida albicans (thrush).	Refer to MDT for treatment.
Dried secretions on hard palate	Buildup of secretions. Reduced fluid intake.	Liaise with nursing staff about oral care.
Halitosis	Lack of oral care. Problems with dentition. Food residue.	Liaise with nursing staff about oral care. Refer to dentist. Recommendations to clear oral cavity of food residue after meals.

Oral care for people unable to carry this out for themselves is a nursing duty. However, if our client with EDS needs presents with any oral care concerns when we assess them, this will affect the results of the assessment and will be causing the client discomfort and possibly embarrassment. As SLTs, we may need therefore to carry out some oral care prior to continuing with assessment. We should use the mouthcare products recommended by the service in which we work. Various products are suitable for clients with EDS needs, such as non-foaming toothpaste, soft toothbrushes and lip moistening gels.

> **O CLINICAL TOP TIP**
>
> Oral care is essential for optimising health but also for maintaining dignity and comfort. This is particularly pertinent at end of life, when clients are unable to eat and drink. Maintaining good oral hygiene may provide relatives with a sense of purpose and of being able to provide a small service to the dying loved-one. Our role is to support them to carry out this care in the optimal way and to help them feel confident.

P IS FOR . . .

POSITIONING

Optimal positioning for safe eating and drinking is to be seated upright, with the head, neck and trunk in midline. Physiotherapy and occupational therapy colleagues can help clients attain and maintain this position. Clients who cannot transfer to a chair may need a profiling bed in order to achieve as upright a position as possible. However, even in a profiling bed, clients can slip down and become semi-reclined, which may necessitate further repositioning. Clients who use a wheelchair may need special adaptations to ensure an upright head and trunk posture, such as a headrest and tray.

A slight chin tuck offers optimal airway protection during eating and drinking.

Safe swallowing recommendations may include suggestions about positioning. An example might be: 'Ensure X is seated upright when eating and drinking. Head, neck and trunk should be in the midline, with the chin tucked down towards the chest.'

If a client is experiencing oral and/or pharyngeal residue post-swallow, we might also recommend that they remain in an upright position for 30 minutes to an hour after eating, so that pooled residue has the opportunity to be swallowed and does not inadvertently enter the pharynx/laryngeal vestibule when the client lies down.

For some clients, however, optimal positioning for eating and drinking is difficult to achieve – for example, because of kyphosis (curvature of the spine), hemiparesis (weakness of one side of the body) or hemiplegia (paralysis of one side of the body). Other patients may have to remain supine or prone in bed for medical or other reasons. Before progressing with clinical assessment and management of the swallow, and for all oral intake, the client should be in as optimal a position as possible. This may mean calling on MDT colleagues such as physiotherapists and nurses to help. Profiling beds, pillows, wheelchair trays and headrests may all be utilised to ensure good positioning. Even with these strategies, optimal positioning may not be achievable, and we may have to proceed with the client in *as optimal position as possible*. There may be some instances where you decide that clinical assessment of the swallow may not proceed to oral trials because the client is in such a poor position for swallowing (eg, someone in a non-profiling bed who is supine and cannot be transferred to a chair). In this instance, we would liaise with the MDT as a matter of urgency to see whether a profiling bed could be provided or repositioning of the client could be prioritised.

Changes in head and body position may also be used therapeutically in order to minimise aspiration (see Table 29).

Try these head/body positions out during VF – this enables you, as the clinician, to check that they are beneficial, and the

Table 29 Therapeutic head and body positions

Head/body position	When is it useful?	Rationale
Chin tuck	Reduced airway protection. Delay in swallow trigger.	Widens the vallecular space and tongue base comes nearer to the pharyngeal wall, narrowing the entrance to the airway.
Head turn to the affected side	Unilateral pharyngeal weakness.	Changes anatomy to effectively close off the weaker side.
Head tilt to the stronger side	Unilateral pharyngeal weakness.	Bolus is encouraged down the stronger side through gravity.
Semi-reclined	Reduced/no anterior-posterior movement of the bolus in the oral stage, with good pharyngeal stage and airway protection.	Bolus arrives at the back of the mouth because of gravity, where the swallow reflex then triggers.

client may feel more motivated to use them having observed their efficacy. Check the evidence base, too!

PRESBYPHAGIA

An individual who is ageing typically with no underlying neurological, structural or behavioural pathology may nevertheless present with some changes to their swallow function (presbyphagia). All stages of the swallow may be affected through age-related muscle weakness (sarcopenia). For example, certain textures may become more difficult to chew or to hold within the oral cavity. The swallow reflex itself may trigger later than in a younger person – that is, the head of the bolus may enter further into the pharynx before the swallow reflex is triggered. Presbyphagia may mean that the person is more at risk of aspiration; reduced pharyngeal contraction may result in residue accumulating in the valleculae and/or the pyriform sinuses, for example, with the resultant possible overspill into the laryngeal vestibule. A delay in the swallow reflex means that material enters the pharynx while the airway is still open – another potential aspiration risk. Older people may already be implementing strategies to make swallowing less problematic, such as avoiding certain consistencies.

If an older person with no underlying pathology seeks an SLT opinion because of a problematic swallow, a thorough clinical assessment should be carried out to rule out any other pathology. Recommendations can then be discussed regarding keeping the three EDS tenets (safety, nutrition/hydration and quality of life) in balance; these may include advice about positioning or bolus size and consistency. However, older people often instinctively know to avoid certain problematic textures or to adopt other strategies (eg, sitting upright, taking smaller sips or slowing down eating).

OSTEOPHYTES

Often occurring in older age and more common in men than in women (Papadopoulou et al, 2013), osteophytes are bony protrusions (or spurs) which can grow from various bones in the human body.

Osteophytes are idiopathic (ie, they have no identifiable cause) and are often non-symptomatic. However, some EDS issues may ensue when osteophytes develop from the anterior cervical vertebrae. Osteophytes typically develop at C5-C6 but may also be seen at the level of C2-C4. The bony spurs may press on the pharynx and/or oesophagus in these areas, causing a change to the anatomy and therefore to the physiology of the swallow. Common complaints include:

- odynophagia (pain on swallowing), because of inflammation around the osteophyte and possible friction against another structure;
- globus or a sensation of something in the throat; and
- aspiration as a result of altered anatomy and physiology, with resultant chest signs – one example of this is a reduction in epiglottic retroversion, resulting in reduced airway protection.

Large osteophytes in this area may cause airway obstruction, stridor (an unusual, often high-frequency respiratory sound caused by a narrowed airway) and obstructive sleep apnoea.

The presence of osteophytes may be suspected after a detailed case history and discussion of symptoms, but conclusive diagnosis must be made via VF. Because bony structures (eg, the mandible) show up so well on X-ray, osteophytes on the anterior vertebrae can be easily visualised during VF, their impact on the swallow process determined and possible management ideas trialled.

Treatment centres on minimising aspiration and discomfort, usually through recommendation of easier-to-manage consistencies. Head positions as a compensatory swallow strategy are not normally recommended because people with anterior osteophytes can have quite a rigid cervical spine with restricted spinal movements, so motion in all planes can be limited. For example, although chin tuck may be useful in some patients for increasing airway protection, a client with anterior osteophytes might be unable to effect the head flexion necessary for this position.

Pain on swallowing and aspiration risk are normally worse on solids than liquids but osteophytes tend to continue to grow, so symptoms may change over time.

Ultimately, surgery may be needed to excise the osteophytes and alleviate the dysphagia symptoms.

PULSE OXIMETRY

Pulse oximetry constitutes one of the instrumental methods of assessing the swallow, but its evidence base is equivocal. A pulse oximeter passes two wavelengths of light through a body part (normally the forefinger but sometimes an earlobe or toe) to a sensor in the device. This measures the amount of infra-red light which has been absorbed by the haemoglobin in the blood. Haemoglobin carries oxygen in the blood, so the figure on the device (the oxygen saturation) refers to the percentage of haemoglobin that is carrying oxygen. The higher the number, the more oxygenated the blood. A typical reading is between 95% and 100%. Readings below 92% are normally considered to be an indication of hypoxaemia (low oxygen levels).

The premise for the use of pulse oximetry as part of the swallow assessment is that if the client aspirates, chest status and breathing will be affected, and oxygen levels will drop. A drop of 2% is considered an indication of reduced pulmonary function. However, a drop in oxygen saturation may also occur as a result of normal apnoea in the pharyngeal stage, as the vocal folds close to protect the airway. Nevertheless, pulse oximetry is relatively affordable, portable, readily available and non-invasive, and as such may contribute to the clinician's overall assessment toolkit. You cannot definitively diagnose aspiration using pulse oximetry, but a drop in oxygen saturation during oral intake *may* be one indicator of an aspiration event.

In an acute hospital, pulse oximeters (often combined with heart rate and blood pressure monitors) are readily available on the ward. If you work out in the community, it might be worth investing in a portable pulse oximeter, to add to your assessment toolkit.

P CLINICAL TOP TIP

The best position for safe swallowing is upright, head, neck and trunk in midline with a slight chin tuck. Encourage your client where possible to eat and drink sitting in a chair at a table looking down at their food.

Q IS FOR . . .

QUESTIONS TO ASK THE CLIENT AND CARER (CASE HISTORY)

The client case history forms an important part of the information-gathering process (along with C for clinical history). Understanding the client's lived experience of a condition or symptom helps to create therapeutic rapport and imbues the clinical encounter with an essence of trust. During the case history interview, try to reflect back the client's own words, to show that you have both listened and understood. For example, if the client complains of 'a feeling of food getting stuck' in their throat, ask them: 'Where does it feel like it is getting stuck?' or 'Can you show me where it feels stuck?'

Ask questions which help in your clinical decision-making, such as those set out in Table 30.

Table 30 Questions to ask the client (case history)

Question	Why are you asking?
Can you describe the difficulty you are having with swallowing?	Listening to the client's concerns helps us to understand their lived experience of the problem.
Did it occur suddenly or gradually?	The clinical history should suggest the cause of the dysphagia (ie, whether it was sudden, as in the case of a stroke, or more gradual, as in neurodegenerative conditions). However, even in sudden onset conditions, there may have been a pre-existing dysphagia.
Has it got any better or worse?	With sudden onset dysphagia, you are likely to see some improvement. In neurodegenerative conditions, the dysphagia will deteriorate over time.

(*Continued*)

Table 30 (Continued)

Question	Why are you asking?
Is your swallowing worse at particular times of day?	Some conditions are affected by fatigue or medication.
Do you have more difficulties swallowing certain consistencies/textures?	Helps us to consider which parts of the swallow physiology are affected and which consistencies to trial during the CSE.
What are you managing to eat and drink at the moment?	Helps us to establish the quantity and consistency of current intake.
Do you need any help to eat and drink?	Needing help to eat and drink means that the oral preparatory stage is affected. Being helped to eat and drink bypasses some key elements of the oral preparatory stage, such as cortical readiness.
Do you experience any pain on swallowing?	Pain on swallowing (odynophagia) may indicate effort or a SOL.
Do you have any chest problems such as asthma or COPD?	Any pre-existing respiratory problems may make the client less able to tolerate any aspiration. We need a baseline of chest status.
Have you had any recent chest infections?	History of chest infections *may* indicate aspiration.
Are you on any medication?	Some medication can affect the EDS process (see M for medication).
Do you have any food allergies or dietary requirements?	To ensure that only appropriate foodstuffs are used in oral trials.
Is there is anything else you would like to say?	A very open final question like this allows the client to tell you anything of note that you may have missed. It affords an opportunity to ask you questions or seek clarification.

There may be some instances when you have to ask for information from the carer or relative rather than the client themselves. For example, your client's level of arousal might be low, they might be very unwell or they may have language or other cognitive difficulties. Some examples of what you might ask a relative are listed in Table 31.

Table 31 Questions to ask the carer

Question	Why are you asking?
When did you first notice a difficulty with their swallowing? Have these difficulties got any worse or better?	In some aetiologies, the onset of dysphagia may be insidious.
What do you notice when they eat or drink?	Encouraging the carer to describe the issues in their own words allows you to mirror their vocabulary.
Do they avoid/do you avoid offering any particular food or drink?	Avoidance may be an indication that the client is anticipating difficulty in swallowing a particular type of food or fluid – the relative may see a pattern.
Do you notice any coughing/wet voice when they eat or drink? If so, are there some textures that cause this more than others?	The carer may be more aware of this than the client themselves.
Do you notice more difficulties at different times of the day?	Carers may see a pattern related to fatigue or medication.
Do you notice them coughing at other times?	Coughing away from mealtimes may indicate post-swallow penetration/ aspiration and/or chest problems.
How are they positioned when they eat/drink?	Gives an indication of whether the client is habitually in an optimal position for safe swallowing or not.
Have they had any recent periods of illness?	If the client has had several trips to the GP in recent weeks and months, it is worth asking explicitly about treatment for chest infections.

You may also want to gather more information by asking pertinent questions of the MDT. Once a clinical history and a case history have been taken, the CSE can begin, based on this information.

Q CLINICAL TOP TIP

Remember that taking the case history may be the first of many clinical encounters with the client – try to make it as therapeutic as possible by employing good active listening skills. Show your interest by leaning forward, holding eye contact and paraphrasing what they say, to indicate that you have both listened and understood correctly. Adopt Rogers' (1951) tenets of empathy, congruence and unconditional positive regard, or van Manen's (2016) ideas of listening to the client with an attitude of openness and awe. Never underestimate the therapeutic power of being listened to!

R IS FOR . . .

RESIDUE

After swallowing, some food or fluid may not enter the oesophagus but may remain in the oral cavity or pharynx.

ORAL RESIDUE

Residue may be found in the anterior and lateral sulci of the oral cavity – that is, between the gum (gingiva) and the inner cheek/bottom lip. Oral residue is more likely if the individual has weakened buccal musculature, poor lingual control and/or reduced intra-oral sensation.

Residue occurs in people with and without EDS needs but is normally managed by effective movement of the tongue to locate and dislodge residue, as well as good clearing swallows.

People with unilateral weakness to the orofacial area and tongue (eg, those who have had a unilateral cortical stroke) may experience oral residue accumulating on the weaker side; reduced buccal tone and reduced tongue movement and strength on the affected side mean that food residue is more likely both to fall into the sulcus and to be more difficult to extricate. Reduced sensation on the affected side may also mean that the client is unaware of the residue.

Oral residue presents a potential risk because any material left in the mouth post-swallow may slip into the pharynx (particularly if the client lies down soon after eating). Residue which has been sitting in the oral cavity may attract bacteria; if this is then aspirated, the risk of a chest infection developing increases.

Oral residue may be assessed by asking the client whether they can feel anything left in the mouth after swallowing. You may also want to look in the oral cavity with a pen torch.

Management strategies include reminding the client to do a sweep of the sulci with their tongue or manually removing the residue. You may want to recommend that the client remain upright for 30 minutes to an hour after mealtimes, to allow for residue to be managed.

PHARYNGEAL RESIDUE

The pharynx contains a number of small pockets of tissue bilaterally into which food or fluid may fall and remain post-swallow. A vallecula is from the Latin for 'small dip' or 'small valley' and the valleculae of the pharynx are formed by mucosa (glossoepiglottic fold) at the base of the epiglottis meeting the base of the tongue. Lower down in the hypopharynx behind the entrance to the laryngeal vestibule lie the pyriform (pear-shaped) fossae (ditches) or sinuses.

The valleculae and pyriform sinuses cannot be seen on clinical examination; an instrumental assessment such as VF or FEES is needed to confirm any suspicions of pharyngeal pooling. Pharyngeal residue may be measured by providing a percentage. For example, in your report you might state something like: '25% of the bolus remained in the valleculae post-swallow.' If unilateral pooling or residue is suspected, an anterior-posterior videofluoroscopic view is useful to visualise asymmetry.

Strategies such as head positions aimed at minimising residue and pooling may also be carried out during the instrumental procedure to check their efficacy. For example, you may want to try a head turn to the affected side if a client has unilateral pharyngeal pooling.

Pharyngeal residue (in either the valleculae or the pyriform sinuses) post-swallow may constitute a risk for the client, as the airway is only closed during the swallow; after the swallow, the vocal and vestibular folds open again so that any material near the laryngeal vestibule may potentially be aspirated.

Management strategies for pharyngeal residue include:

- a second clearing swallow on each bolus;
- forced expiration post-swallow to move residue further up into the pharynx, followed by a second swallow;

- head turn to the affected side;
- head tilt to the unaffected side;
- effortful swallow;
- supraglottic swallow; and
- super-supraglottic swallow.

RISK

Everything that we do in life carries a certain level of risk: we take a risk when we cross the road or take a plane. As adults, we weigh up those risks before deciding on a course of action. The language of dysphagia often centres on safety (or lack thereof) and risk; we talk about safe swallowing strategies or the client being unsafe for any oral intake. However, the risk/safety concept is not straightforward: a poor swallow *may* mean that the individual is more susceptible to chest infections, but poor nutrition and hydration and low quality of life are also risks to physical and mental health. The biomedical ethical principle of non-maleficence (Beauchamp and Childress, 1979) does not simply refer to avoidance of aspiration risk at all costs. Beneficence and non-maleficence also include finding solutions which are acceptable to the client and as beneficial to their physical and mental health as possible.

The language of risk can be quite frightening and also somehow transfers the onus of responsibility onto the client. Hence, a client who has been deemed 'unsafe on all oral intake' but who continues to eat and drink regardless is often made to sign a disclaimer, stating that they are aware of the risks. They are sometimes labelled as 'non-compliant' – another unhelpful term to be avoided in person-centred and compassionate care. More helpful in this scenario, I think, is to coach the client in the changes in the swallow, the potential effect that these could have on their ability to eat and drink and the possible adverse reactions (eg, coughing and potentially becoming unwell); and then to decide together on the best way forward. For example, is there a head position, manoeuvre or adaptive utensil which makes the swallow safer and is acceptable to them?

Eating and drinking with acknowledged risk has become accepted practice in an effort to give clients the autonomy to take risks in relation to their eating and drinking and to encourage clinicians to become more risk-enabling (Hansjee, 2018; Hansjee et al, 2021). This may be, for example, because they are approaching the end of their life and avoiding aspiration becomes rather pointless – the quality of life tenet has become the primary of the three.

As clinicians, we cannot be risk averse in EDS assessment and management. As the principal clinician in dysphagia, we need to be able to push the client to the limits of what they can manage. If we do not do this, clients run the risk of eating and drinking consistencies or implementing certain strategies that are not necessary, but which may impact quality of life. We are constantly weighing up risk versus benefit in assessment and management choices. For example, do the benefits of the results of VF outweigh the risks of ionising radiation and possible discomfort? Do the potential benefits of no longer having to have thickened fluids outweigh the possible risks of assessing someone on thin fluids?

R CLINICAL TOP TIP

The language of risk is perhaps an unhelpful one for clients who are keen to continue eating and drinking as normally as possible for as long as possible. Maybe we should reframe this by talking about minimising discomfort and possible health-related consequences of eating and drinking?

S IS FOR . . .

SESSION PLANNING

Creating a session plan for all our SLT interventions allows us to think deeply about the rationale and evidence base for the intervention, as well as the practicalities of what resources are needed, how long activities are expected to take and how we might make the activities easier or more difficult, depending on how the client is performing. Session-planning is a particularly useful discipline when we are students or new to a clinical area.

A good session plan comprises the following:

- client details (name, date of birth, ward/facility);
- long-term goal (often this is set by the client themselves);
- short-term goals (set collaboratively between the client and the SLT);
- session goal;
- activities;
- step-up and step-down activities;
- resources needed;
- time for each activity; and
- evidence base for intervention.

Table 32 may be used as a template for planning an EDS session with a client.

Table 32 EDS session plan

Client name:	Date of birth:		Ward/location:	
Date:	Time:			
Client's long-term EDS goal:				
Short-term goal(s):				
Session goal(s):				
Activity/ies:	Time	Resources	Step-up	Step-down
Evidence base:				
Reflection on session:				

> **S CLINICAL TOP TIP**
>
> Drawing up a session plan is intrinsic to developing our clinical reasoning, encouraging us to consider why we have chosen this particular intervention for this particular client. How does this intervention relate to the results of their assessment and what is the evidence for its efficacy?

T IS FOR . . .

TASTES FOR PLEASURE

Some clients may be temporarily or permanently unable to take food and drink orally and instead rely on enteral feeding to derive all their nutrition and hydration. For quality-of-life purposes, it may be possible to offer small tastes for pleasure – that is, very small amounts of food or drink which provide the taste but, because of the small quantity, do not pose too much of an aspiration risk. These tastes should, of course, be ones that the client likes or has requested, and should be of a consistency which does not constitute a choking hazard – for example, a tiny amount of yoghurt or a favourite pudding may be appropriate. If tastes for pleasure are to be implemented, part of the management plan should be monitoring of chest status.

Small tastes may also constitute part of a therapy plan (see taste stimulation under D for direct therapy techniques).

THREE TENETS OF EDS MANAGEMENT

In setting EDS goals and planning management with our adult clients, three important tenets must be considered (MacKenzie, 2024):

- safety;
- nutrition and hydration; and
- quality of life.

For example, although we have concerns about a client aspirating (safety), we cannot ignore their desire to continue to eat and drink orally (quality of life) or their physical need to do so (nutrition and hydration).

DOI: 10.4324/9781003480877-20

In different scenarios, the three tenets may be in disequilibrium. For example, for a person with a lifelong EDS need – such as a person with cerebral palsy – quality of life may take precedence. For someone with a temporary dysphagia – such as an individual undergoing a limited period of radiotherapy for head and neck cancer – safety might trump the others. For someone who is physically weak and at risk of malnutrition and skin breakdown, nutrition and hydration supersede safety of the swallow and quality of life.

It is a good idea to keep the three tenets in mind when you are discussing and planning therapy goals. You may have separate goals which relate to each tenet.

Sometimes there is an uneasy tension between the three and this is discussed in more detail under R for risk.

TRACHEOSTOMY

Student speech and language therapists and newly qualified practitioners are expected to have some knowledge of EDS assessment and management of clients with a tracheostomy tube in situ, although independent care of these clients will only be undertaken with post-registration training and/or experience.

A tracheostomy tube may be sited (in a surgical procedure known as a 'tracheotomy') either as an emergency (eg, in a client with severe trauma) or as a planned procedure (eg, in a client undergoing extensive surgery for head and neck cancer). Either way, the tracheostomy allows the client to breathe when normal respiration is compromised. The surgeon creates a hole in the anterior neck, between the second and third tracheal rings below the level of the vocal folds, and a tube is inserted into the hole, creating a direct pathway from the anterior neck to the trachea. This allows air to flow in and out of the trachea and lungs directly through the hole (stoma) in the anterior neck. Unlike a stoma created in a laryngectomy patient, the tracheostoma must have a tube in it to remain patent; when the tubing is removed, the stoma will close.

Because air now flows directly from the lungs through the bronchi and trachea and out of the neck stoma before reaching the vocal folds, voicing is no longer possible for clients with a tracheostomy; however, some adaptations to the tracheostomy tube can facilitate voicing. To enable the client to voice, a speaking valve may be attached to the end of an uncuffed tracheostomy tube. This one-way valve allows inspired air in but shuts off on expiration, thereby redirecting the air up through the vocal folds, the pharynx and the articulators. A speaking valve may also be used in the process of weaning a client off the tracheostomy, as it allows for more normality of breathing (as far as exhalation is concerned), so acts as a bridge between tracheostomy breathing and oral/nasal breathing. In terms of swallowing, the speaking valve starts to renormalise the pressures within the pharynx.

Humidification of inhaled air is also problematic; the air in no longer warmed or filtered by mucous, cilia and blood vessels in the nose. Humidification and filtering are provided artificially by attaching a heat and moisture exchange (HME) device to the tracheostomy tube, known as a 'Swedish nose'. This is comprised of spongy material which absorbs moisture from exhaled air and releases it back into inhaled air. Without a HME, secretions may become thick and block the tracheostomy tube and patients may be more prone to infection. A Swedish nose is designed not to be locked onto the tracheostomy tube; if the client coughs, it will fly off. For hygiene purposes, it should be replaced every 24 hours.

The tracheostomy tube is secured by a flange with straps which tie around the neck, to stop the tube from becoming displaced. Most tracheostomy tubes comprise an outer tube or cannula which stays in the stoma and an inner cannula which can be periodically removed, washed and replaced into the outer cannula. This is normally a nursing task but may fall to the SLT to do if the cannula needs cleaning before an SLT session can continue.

Inner and outer cannulae may have one small hole or multiple holes at the bend of the tube. Known as 'fenestration' (from the Latin for 'window'), this allows some air to travel up through the vocal folds on expiration, thereby enabling voicing to occur. Fenestration may also be advocated in EDS to allow more normalisation of subglottic pressure.

A tracheostomy tube may also be cuffed – that is, there is a small balloon around the part of the tube which sits in the trachea. When inflated with air from a syringe via a pilot balloon attached to the flange, the cuff creates a seal between the tracheal wall and the lumen of the tracheostomy tube. With an inflated cuff in situ, no air can travel up past the tracheostomy tube and through the vocal folds, so voicing is not possible. Individuals who require ventilator support for respiration will have a cuffed tracheostomy in situ. Before the cuff is deflated for any reason (eg, a change of tube), any aspirate must be suctioned off from the top of the cuff via an above-cuff suction device; otherwise, material which has gathered on top of the cuff will travel further down into the trachea and eventually to the lungs. Suction is usually carried out by a nurse or physiotherapist; you should not carry out tracheal suction yourself unless you have had specific training.

Table 33 The potential impact of the presence of a tracheostomy tube on the swallow process

Issue	Potential effect on the swallow	Reason	Evidence
Reduced hyolaryngeal excursion	Reduced airway protection.	Physical proximity of tube anchors the larynx.	Amathieu et al, 2012
Change to subglottic pressure	Material may remain in the airway.	Stoma creates change in pressure.	Gross, Mahlmann and Grayhack, 2003
Reduced cough reflex	Reduced airway protection, silent aspiration.	Larynx and pharynx become desensitised.	Park and Lee, 2018
Reduced efficacy of taste receptors	Altered taste.	Lack of airflow through the nose reduces sense of smell (anosmia). Smell and taste are closely related, so taste may also be affected.	Tsikoudas, Barnes and White, 2011

A cuffed tracheostomy is sometimes considered as a way of preventing aspiration; however, the tracheal wall-tracheostomy tube seal is never complete, so aspirate can still seep past the cuff.

An artificially created hole in the neck is likely to affect the swallow process. Table 33 outlines some of the potential EDS difficulties associated with the presence of a tracheostomy tube.

DECANNULATION

Sometimes a person may require a tracheostomy forever or for the foreseeable future. For others, the tracheostomy is a temporary measure to help with respiration and the plan may be to remove the tracheostomy in a process known as 'decannulation'. The SLT is an intrinsic member of the decannulation team. Table 34 sets out a suggested decannulation protocol.

Table 34 The decannulation process

Decannulation step	MDT member	Rationale
Decision to decannulate	All – final decision by medic	All factors to be considered.
Above-cuff suction	Nurse/respiratory physiotherapist	Removal of any potential aspirate lying on the cuff to prevent this from falling further into trachea on deflation.
Cuff deflation	Nurse/respiratory physiotherapist	To minimise possibility of tethering of larynx. Allows some air to flow up around the tube.
Change to cuffless tracheostomy	Nurse/medic	To minimise possibility of tethering of larynx. Allows some air to flow up around the tube.
Change to fenestrated tracheostomy	Nurse/medic	To allow air up through the glottis (cough). Normalises sub-glottic and glottic pressure.

(*Continued*)

Table 34 (Continued)

Decannulation step	MDT member	Rationale
Trials of finger occlusion	SLT	Temporarily allows for coughing and normalises pressures. Creates temporary closed respiratory system. Client can safely practise coordination of breathing and voicing/coughing.
Trials of speaking valve	SLT	One-way valve allows air in through the tracheostomy tube during inspiration but closes and redirects air up through glottis on expiration. Allows voicing and coughing, and normalises pressure. Creates temporary closed respiratory system.
Trials of capping off	SLT/nurse	Mimics decannulation. Allows MDT to determine whether client can cope without tracheostomy. Creates temporary closed respiratory system.
Removal of tracheostomy tube	Nurse/medic	Creates permanent closed respiratory system.

Once the tracheostomy tube has been removed, the stoma should close without any need for stitches.

EDS assessment and intervention with tracheostomised clients should also take into account other co-occurring considerations which may impact swallowing, such as neurological or structural issues.

EDS ASSESSMENT

Assessment of the tracheostomised client broadly takes the same form as that used with a non-tracheostomised client: both a CSE and instrumental assessment technique may be utilised.

Information-gathering will include details outlined under C for clinical history, but may also include the following:

- the reason for the tracheostomy;
- the length of time for which the tracheostomy has been in situ;
- the type of tracheostomy tube (ie, cuffed/uncuffed, fenestrated/unfenestrated); and
- any trials of a speaking valve.

Case history-taking may be more problematic with the tracheostomised client; if voicing is not possible, a simple pen and paper or electronic tablet may be enough to facilitate their ability to answer. However, there may of course be other reasons why answering questions is difficult for the tracheostomised client, such as low level of arousal or cognitive and/or language challenges. As with other client groups, you may need to adapt your language or take a case history from the next of kin (see under Q for questions to ask the client and carer).

Laryngeal palpation may not be possible with this client group, or finger placement may have to be adapted to accommodate the tube.

Oral trials may be attempted with the tracheostomised client (depending on the results of the rest of the CSE). However, you will need to take into account the possible detrimental effects of the presence of the tube on swallow anatomy and physiology and mitigate these effects (see Table 35).

Table 35 How to mitigate potential issues resulting from the presence of the tracheostomy tube

Potential issue	Mitigation
Tethering/anchoring of the larynx, impeding hyolaryngeal excursion	Cuff deflation or cuffless tracheostomy tube.
Reduced sub-glottic and glottic pressure	Use of one-way speaking valve or occlusion of the tracheostomy tube with decannulation cap.
Altered taste	Trials of different foodstuffs.

An additional assessment technique used exclusively with tracheostomised clients – for reasons which will become obvious – is the Modified Evans Blue Dye Test (MEBDT). This assessment technique has peaked and waned in popularity over the years, but research suggests that the MEBDT can at least identify people without oropharyngeal dysphagia even if its ability correctly to identify presence of dysphagia is more equivocal (Béchet et al, 2016).

The procedure is predicated on the understanding that if material is aspirated, it can be suctioned out of the trachea in a tracheostomised patient. Blue dye is placed on the client's tongue and the client is instructed to swallow. Immediately after the swallow, the nurse or physiotherapist suctions via the tracheostomy tube. If any saliva has been aspirated, the suction catheter should contain blue-stained sputum. The nurse or physiotherapist may also suction a few minutes or hours later to check for further aspiration or aspiration of pooled secretions. The blue dye test is notorious for providing false negatives but may detect gross aspiration. Even if aspiration is proven, however, the MEBDT does not help the clinician determine why it has occurred, and a more reliable instrumental assessment may be warranted.

VF and FEES may both be used on the tracheostomised client; portable FEES may be particularly useful for clients who are unwell and need to remain in bed, or who are unable to be brought to the X-ray suite.

EDS MANAGEMENT

Oral intake may be reintroduced in a person with a tracheostomy; all oral trials, however, must take place with the cuff down or with a cuffless tracheostomy tube in situ. Other management strategies may also be appropriate, such as texture modification or stimulation techniques. Head positions and manoeuvres may be more problematic because of the presence of the tube.

KEY EDS DIFFERENCES BETWEEN TRACHEOSTOMY AND LARYNGECTOMY

Although a client who has undergone a laryngectomy and a client with a tracheostomy may look superficially similar (ie, there is a visible opening in the neck), the differences in anatomy are key to understanding the differences in EDS assessment and management. In the case of tracheostomy, basic anatomy remains unchanged, except that there is now a direct route for air from the trachea to outside the body. In laryngectomy, anatomy is drastically altered, with the oesophagus and trachea no longer sharing a common entrance (in the form of the pharynx).

In tracheostomy, potential EDS difficulties relate to the mechanical presence of the tube, as well as to the new aperture. In laryngectomy, EDS difficulties relate mostly to the surgically created fistula between the oesophageal and tracheal walls, as well as possible problems with reflux as a result of the cricopharyngeal sphincter being removed. Aspiration in a tracheostomised patient is possible because of the proximity of the respiratory and digestive systems. Aspiration in a laryngectomy patient is possible not because the two systems are linked (they no longer are), but because of the surgically placed fistula in which the voice prosthesis is placed. If you look under A for aetiology (structural), you will see why aspiration may occur through the fistula and how we can help prevent it.

T CLINICAL TOP TIP

As the SLT in the MDT, you may be asked your advice about whether decannulation should commence from an SLT perspective. As a rule of thumb, both speaking and swallowing will always be enhanced by removal of the tracheostomy tube.

U IS FOR . . .

UVULA

From the Latin for 'little grape', the uvula is the small structure protruding from the back edge of the velum (soft palate). The velum and uvula rise up together to meet Passavant's ridge on the posterior pharyngeal wall in order to achieve velopharyngeal closure at the point of swallow. The uvula is comprised of connective tissue, muscle and serous glands which produce saliva, thereby contributing to the oral preparatory stage of swallowing. The muscle within the uvula is called the 'musculus uvulae' and its function is to shorten and broaden the uvula, contributing (with the velum) to the closure of the nasopharynx. It is governed by CN X (vagus). If velopharyngeal closure is compromised, clients may experience nasal regurgitation or food/fluid entering the nasal cavity (and sometimes exiting from the nose). Nasal regurgitation is not harmful *per se* but may be very unpleasant and embarrassing for the individual.

Occasionally, people can be born with a cleft (bifid or bifurcated) uvula, which usually contains less muscle and may be less effective at helping to create velopharyngeal closure during the swallow.

Uvulitis may ensue if the mucous membrane of the uvula is inflamed. As the tissue swells and touches the tongue or the pharyngeal wall, the gag reflex may be elicited and the person may experience a very unpleasant sensation of choking.

U CLINICAL TOP TIP

If you place a tongue depressor on the client's tongue and use a pen torch to look inside the oral cavity, you will see the uvula hanging down at the back of the mouth with the faucial arches either side of it. Ask your client to produce /ɑ/ and you will see both the velum and the uvula rise up.

V IS FOR . . .

VIDEOFLUOROSCOPY (VF)

WHAT IS IT?

Referred to in the literature as the 'gold standard' (Logemann, 1996) of swallowing assessment, VF is an instrumental, objective method of visualising the anatomy and physiology of the swallow process, from the oral preparatory stage to the oesophageal stage.

VF uses real-time moving images in the form of X-rays to show the path of the bolus from entry to the oral cavity through to its journey down the oesophagus by peristalsis – that is, the entire physiology of the swallow process. This enables the clinician to determine where in the process problems might occur and, more importantly in terms of managing the difficulty, why.

VF is sometimes referred to as a 'modified barium swallow'; the procedure grew out of one that focused on the gastrointestinal tract (eg, when diagnosing stomach ulcers). The videofluoroscopic study of the swallow focuses much more on the head and neck, so that the oral preparatory, oral and pharyngeal stages can all be visualised.

Images may be taken in the lateral plane, the anterior-posterior plane or both, depending on what the clinician wants to see. For example, if asymmetry is suspected, an anterior-posterior view will allow the clinician to confirm this.

WHAT HAPPENS DURING THE PROCEDURE?

The client is positioned upright (either seated or standing) and a C-arm is positioned around them – this is a medical imaging device which comprises an X-ray source and detector. Because the C-arm can be moved around the client, people who use a wheelchair can be comfortably seated and the C-arm can move around them. If the client's seating system includes a metal headrest, this may need to be removed; otherwise, it will obscure the image. If the client is ambulant, they can either stand for the procedure or sit upright in a chair.

The client must be fully alert for the procedure. They also need a reasonable level of language and cognition – for example, they will need to be able to understand and remember instructions such as: 'Take a mouthful and hold it in your mouth until I say, "Swallow."'

Various consistencies may be trialled, depending on the client's clinical presentation. Often, the referring clinician will request the consistencies to be trialled, as well as any possible management strategies. All clients should have had a clinical assessment prior to referral for VF, with clear objectives for the procedure outlined. For example, it may be that the referring clinician suspects silent aspiration; or they may want to see whether a certain head position minimises aspiration.

Food and drink are mixed with a radio-opaque contrast material, such as barium sulphate, so that it shows up on the X-ray. If a solid consistency is to be trialled, the barium can be spread on the food like a paste. The bolus and bone generally show as dark in the images, with air being white, although this can be reversed. VF (and FEES) are sometimes referred to as 'objective' assessments, which relates to the fact that certain measurements can be taken during the procedure. Although still necessitating a certain degree of subjectivity, these encourage consensus or near-consensus between clinicians. Common measurements taken during VF are outlined in Table 36.

A common way of quantifying the presence and amount of penetration and/or aspiration is an eight-point scale of severity called the Penetration/Aspiration Scale (Rosenbek et al, 1996) (see table 37). One on the scale indicates no evidence of aspiration or penetration, while eight indicates that material is entering the trachea with no attempt by the client to clear (ie, silent aspiration).

Table 36 Common measurements taken during VF

	What is it?	How do we measure it?
Oral transit time	Time taken from commencement of the oral phase (ie, the anterior-posterior transference of the bolus) to the passing of the leading edge of the bolus across the point where the mandible crosses the tongue base (ramus).	Images can be viewed frame by frame. Transit times can be measured in milliseconds (msecs).
Pharyngeal transit time	Time taken from the swallow triggering to the tail of the bolus passing through the cricopharyngeal sphincter.	Images can be viewed frame by frame. Transit times can be measured in msecs.
Level of swallow trigger	Level reached by the head of the bolus when the swallow reflex is triggered.	The landmark reached at the point of trigger (eg, the valleculae).
Penetration and aspiration	Material entering the laryngeal vestibule/passing through the vocal folds.	Penetration/Aspiration Scale (Rosenbek et al, 1996).
Residue	Food/fluid left over after a swallow has occurred.	Estimate of percentage of original bolus.
Presence/ absence of cough	Reflex to eject material from the laryngeal vestibule back into the pharynx.	Observation of cough if/when laryngeal penetration/ aspiration occurs.

Table 37 Based on Rosenbek's Penetration/Aspiration Scale (1996).

Score	Penetration/ aspiration	Description
1	None	Material does not enter the larynx or trachea.
2	Penetration	Material enters the laryngeal vestibule but there are attempts to clear.
3	Penetration	Material enters the laryngeal vestibule but there are no attempts to clear.
4	Penetration	Material contacts the true vocal folds and there are attempts to clear.
5	Penetration	Material contacts the true vocal folds and there are no attempts to clear.

(*Continued*)

Table 37 (Continued)

Score	Penetration/aspiration	Description
6	Aspiration	Material goes past the level of the vocal folds, enters the trachea but is spontaneously cleared back into the larynx or pharynx.
7	Aspiration	Material goes past the level of the vocal folds, enters the trachea and is not cleared despite attempts to do so.
8	Aspiration	Material goes past the level of the vocal folds, enters the trachea and there are no attempts to clear.

Residue may be judged visuo-perceptually as either absent or present, and the anatomical site of any residue can be determined. For example, vallecular residue may be in evidence post swallow. Clinicians may also estimate the amount of the original bolus which remains post swallow and state it as a percentage of the original bolus. Of note is that the viscosity and coating properties of some contrast material may result in over-interpretation of post-swallow residue.

WHY MIGHT YOU REFER A CLIENT?

You might refer a client for an instrumental assessment such as VF if the results of the clinical swallow examination are equivocal. Although we can assess most of the oral preparatory and oral stages clinically, pharyngeal stage issues are far more difficult to gauge at bedside. For example, the point at which the swallow reflex triggers may be estimated during a clinical examination, but only a VF will tell you exactly where the head of the bolus is when the swallow is triggered. Clinicians may suspect a delay in the swallow reflex at bedside, but this can only be diagnosed definitively by watching the progress of the bolus during VF.

Silent aspiration can also only be diagnosed during VF and FEES. Although you may suspect silent aspiration (eg, the client has numerous chest infections with no or few clinical signs of aspiration), it can only be confirmed when aspiration is seen and no cough occurs.

You may want to test out some safer swallowing strategies during VF to see whether they do indeed benefit the client. For example, you could trial different head positions during VF to determine which one helps to minimise aspiration or laryngeal penetration. The client can also see the efficacy (or not) of various positions or manoeuvres, which may help them to understand the rationale for implementing the strategy and increase motivation for doing so.

VF may also be therapeutic in explaining swallow function to clients. For example, someone with dysphagia as a result of a functional neurological disorder may be reassured by objectively observing the safety of their swallow.

PROS AND CONS

VF is a powerful diagnostic tool which provides a comprehensive view of the entire swallow process in real time, from the opening and closing of the mouth to mastication and manipulation of the oral preparatory phase, the tongue's stripping action of the oral phase and the swallow reflex itself at the pharyngeal stage. It may be the instrumental assessment of choice for testing out safer swallowing strategies, diagnosing silent aspiration and supplying the client with biofeedback.

However, VF is not without its disadvantages. The client may feel some discomfort and inconvenience – for example, ingested barium may cause constipation or diarrhoea. VF necessitates exposure to a degree of ionising radiation, with its inherent risks. Aspiration of the contrast material may occur but can be mitigated by calling on the respiratory physiotherapist to implement some chest drainage techniques.

Powerful as it can prove to be as an assessment, not all our clients are suitable candidates for VF. For example, low level of consciousness, medical instability, poor cognition and language levels may all preclude a procedure such as this. In order to undergo VF, clients must also be able to be transported to the X-ray suite, so those who are unable to be transferred from the bed to a chair or wheelchair would not be suitable candidates. Despite best efforts, some clients cannot be positioned in a way that allows for all the anatomy to be visualised, such as people with severe kyphosis.

PERSONNEL

The SLT normally leads the VF clinic, but other members of the team play key roles, as outlined in Table 38.

Table 38 VF personnel and their roles

Team member	Role
SLT	Decides on: • bolus consistency; • bolus size; • plane (lateral or anterior-posterior); • positioning; and • strategies. May give the bolus to the client. Signals to the radiographer when to screen. Reassures the client and gives instructions. Talks through images with the client. Examines images and writes a report based on findings. Liaises with the radiologist, if necessary.
Radiographer	Operates imaging equipment. Liaises with the SLT in terms of where, when and how often to screen. Oversees safety (of the client and all clinic personnel). Liaises with the radiologist if necessary.
SLT assistant/student	Prepares boluses with chosen contrast material.
Carer	May bring familiar food, drink and utensils from home. May be present to reassure the client.
Physiotherapist	May help with positioning the client. May be present (or a bleep away) should aspiration occur.
Radiologist	May be present or available to view images, if necessary.

CONSENT

We must gain and document informed consent for every assessment and intervention carried out with our clients. In the case of VF, careful consideration must be given as to how the client can be best informed. This includes explaining what happens during the procedure, the benefits and risks, how the results will be conveyed and what impact these will have on the management of their eating and drinking. As an SLT, you will use your skills to ensure that all steps of the procedure have been understood – for example, by using pictures, diagrams, gestures and writing key words – and that the client has been empowered to ask questions.

It is best practice to talk through the procedure with the client and gain their consent when you refer them to the VF clinic and then to check consent again when they arrive for the procedure.

As with any consent-gaining, you may need to check for capacity to consent, according to the Mental Capacity Act, 2005.

SAFETY CONSIDERATIONS

VF uses ionising radiation, so it is not a procedure to be taken lightly. We must be sure that the risks of the procedure are outweighed by the potential benefits. How will management of the client (the safety of their swallow, nutrition and hydration and quality of life) be influenced?

The risks of ionising radiation must be mitigated by the implementation of safety measures for the client, any attending carer and all clinic personnel.

The client must be comfortably positioned and have the risks and benefits of the procedure explained to them. The SLT will be moving around the client, handing them utensils and cups or helping them to eat and drink, so they will need to wear protective clothing in the form of a lead apron, thyroid shield and lead gauntlet. Any personnel who do not need to be in the main body of the clinic (eg, the radiographer, students and carer) will stand behind the lead shield. Lead has a high density and atomic number and protects from scattered X-rays in the room.

Personnel (including SLTs) who regularly attend VF clinics should also wear a dosimeter: a small device which measures the amount of ionising radiation that a person has been exposed to over time. Radiation from VF is relatively low compared to other procedures; nevertheless, you should be guided by the radiographer as to how often the client is screened. They may caution you not to carry out multiple repetitions of bolus trials.

Pregnancy does not necessarily preclude being in the VF clinic; however, pregnancy should always be discussed with the radiographer and local recommendations and procedures followed. You may decide not to take part in VF clinics while pregnant if another SLT is available. If the client is pregnant, you might want to consider other instrumental assessment choices, such as FEES.

WRITING THE REPORT

The SLT, radiographer and radiologist (or a combination of these) will interpret the VF images after the procedure and then draw up a written report which can be sent to the referring SLT and any other interested parties (eg, the consultant, GP or nurse). Report templates will vary from service to service but are often structured around the four stages of the swallow, describing what happened at each one with each bolus. At each stage, the components of that stage may be described, such as lip closure during the oral stage or epiglottic retroversion at the pharyngeal stage. As with other SLT reports, a diagnosis and recommendations for further treatment are essential. The Modified Barium Swallow Impairment Profile™ offers a comprehensive and logical report structure.

V CLINICAL TOP TIP

The X-ray suite can be very intimidating, housing lots of medical equipment and machinery. You might want to consider preparing your client prior to the appointment by showing them pictures of the clinic room and of the clinicians wearing lead aprons and thyroid shields.

For some clients (eg, those with a learning disability), a visit to the clinic room prior to the actual appointment may be advisable.

It is the job of all personnel in the clinic to reassure the client and make them feel as comfortable as possible during the procedure.

W IS FOR. . .

WATER – PROTOCOLS AND TESTS

FRAZIER FREE WATER PROTOCOL

The Frazier Free Water Protocol (often abbreviated to the 'Free Water Protocol') was devised in 2005 by Kathy Panther. In 2017, Gillman, Winkler and Taylor conducted a systematic review which concluded that implementing the protocol did not result in aspiration pneumonia in carefully selected adults with EDS needs.

Clients with dysphagia who have been deemed unsafe for oral intake – and are therefore nil by mouth – or those with a compromised swallow who have been recommended thickened fluids may be at risk of dehydration because of reduced fluid intake. Complications of dehydration can be severe, including kidney issues, impaired cognition, urinary tract infections, sepsis and even death.

Aspiration is a prerequisite for aspiration pneumonia; however, not all aspiration results in aspiration pneumonia. Oral and pharyngeal bacteria may, for example, increase the risk of aspirated material triggering aspiration pneumonia. Langmore et al's (1998) seminal article states the other risk factors for development of aspiration pneumonia – namely pre-existing lung problems (eg, COPD), history of smoking, polypharmacy, frailty and reduced mobility.

Clients who are nil by mouth (Hepper et al, 2024) or who are drinking thickened fluids (Swan et al, 2015) report a reduction in their wellbeing and quality of life. Thickened fluids can be so unpalatable to some people that they refuse the recommendation to alter the consistency of their drinks.

The aim of the Free Water Protocol, therefore, is to increase hydration as safely as possible, thus also enhancing quality of life. The premise of the Frazier Free Water Protocol is that clean (ie, not containing harmful bacteria) water – if aspirated – is unlikely to cause chest complications. Small amounts of aspirated water can be reabsorbed back into the body via the aquaporins from the lungs.

The Protocol may be recommended for those who are nil by mouth or those who have been prescribed thickened fluids (Panther, 2005). Thin fluids are offered between meals (at least 30 minutes after mealtimes, to minimise the possibility of food residue in the oral cavity or pharynx being inadvertently washed down), and after assiduous oral care (to minimise bacteria in the oral cavity). Clients may not be suitable for the Protocol if they exhibit impulsive behaviour or excessive coughing on thin fluids, or if their arousal level is low.

TIMED WATER SWALLOW TEST (TWST)

The Timed Water Swallow Test (TWST) (Hughes and Wiles, 1996) involves asking the client to drink either 100 or 150 millilitres of water from a cup as normally as possible. The number of swallows and total time taken to finish the drink are recorded, as well as clinical signs of laryngeal penetration such as a change in voice quality (wet voice) and coughing.

The TWST is very simple to administer and can detect gross aspiration. If aspiration occurs, clean, thin (ie not artificially thickened) water is the substance least likely to cause chest complications. However, the TWST should not be used on clients who have overt oromotor difficulties or a low level of arousal. For these clients, it is obvious from these other signs that aspiration is likely.

The TWST is very much a screening tool and does not allow for a detailed analysis of where breakdown of the swallow process may be happening or what management strategies might be beneficial.

> **W CLINICAL TOP TIP**
>
> Pure water is the substance least likely to cause chest complications if aspirated and can be reabsorbed into the body. If you are tempted to use thickened water in either your assessment or recommendations, don't forget that this can be particularly unpalatable.

X IS FOR . . .

XEROSTOMIA, SIALORRHOEA AND SALIVATION

Saliva is produced by three major sets of salivary glands:

- parotid;
- submandibular; and
- sublingual.

The parotid glands are located just below the ears, the submandibular below the jaw and the sublingual below the tongue in the floor of the mouth. You will remember that the uvula also has the ability to secrete some saliva, as does the oral mucosa of the lips, inner cheeks, hard palate and velum – these are sometimes referred to as the 'minor salivary glands'.

The body produces two different types of saliva: serous (which is watery) and mucous (which has more viscosity).

Serous saliva contains water and a digestive protein enzyme called amylase which can break down starchy materials (as an aside, if fluid is thickened with a starch-based thickening agent, saliva from the rim of the cup can mix with the fluid and the amylase may start to break down that starchy material, thereby creating two different consistencies of fluid). The parotid glands are the main producers of serous saliva.

The submandibular salivary glands secrete both serous and mucous saliva. The sublingual glands produce mostly mucous saliva, which comprises a lubricant-type protein called 'mucin'.

The salivary glands receive innervation from the autonomic nervous system (both sympathetic and parasympathetic). The parotid glands are supplied by CN IX (glossopharyngeal) and the submandibular and sublingual by CN VII (facial). Production of saliva can be stimulated by the taste and feel of the bolus in the mouth, but also by the cognitive process of thinking about eating. Even at rest with no apparent stimulation, saliva is still being produced.

Secretion of saliva is vital to the EDS process (as well as speech – producing phonemes is difficult with a dry mouth):

- Mucous-type saliva acts as a lubricant, combining with food to form a cohesive bolus and allowing the bolus to glide over oral and pharyngeal structures.
- Saliva – being mostly comprised of water – helps to wash away build-up of food residue on the teeth or oral mucosa.
- Saliva has anti-bacterial properties which help to keep the oral cavity clean.

During the oral preparatory stage of the swallow, food is masticated and manipulated with the tongue and saliva is added to create the bolus. Saliva, food and fluid are all kept in the mouth through a combination of lip seal and buccal tension. If lip seal is reduced, saliva may escape anteriorly. If buccal tension is reduced, saliva may fall into the lateral sulci. Continual swallowing throughout the day (and, less so, the night) clears the oral cavity of excess saliva. If the oral preparatory phase is effectively bypassed by the person being helped to eat and drink by someone else, saliva production may be impacted. A strategy here might be to talk to the person about what they are about to taste, as well as allowing them to see and smell the food.

XEROSTOMIA

Xerostomia or dry mouth can have a major effect on EDS, physical health and quality of life. It can be caused by habitual mouth-breathing, certain medications (eg, some antihistamines and antidepressants) or radiation to the salivary glands during radiotherapy for head and neck cancer.

Radiation damage to the salivary glands is permanent, so survivors of head and neck cancer may be left with the distressing after-effects of dry mouth for the rest of their lives. SLT intervention in this instance comprises support and advice on strategies to help counteract the xerostomia. For example, the client may be helped by regular sips of fluid or ice chips, or they may want to avoid very dry foods. Various brands of artificial saliva are also available. Because of the natural cleansing property of saliva, clients with xerostomia may need specific advice regarding oral hygiene.

People who have undergone radiotherapy to the head and neck may experience a change in the consistency of their saliva as opposed to a dry mouth. Thicker saliva is also detrimental to the swallow process and may affect the client's ability to create a bolus. Good fluid intake (particularly regular sips during mealtimes) as well as artificial saliva may also be appropriate for these clients. Make sure you stay up to date with new products which may enter the market and benefit the client.

SIALORRHOEA

The opposite of xerostomia is sialorrhoea, when too much saliva is produced – usually as a side effect of medication, such as some antipsychotics. Sialorrhoea may result in anterior escape of saliva during the oral preparatory and oral stages, which can be distressing for the individual. Excess saliva may also be aspirated prior to a swallow if it enters the pharynx and larynx and the airway is unprotected. However, it is worth remembering that sometimes anterior escape of saliva and/or aspiration of saliva results from a reduced number of spontaneous swallows rather than overproduction of saliva. In this instance, we might refer to the client being unable to manage their own secretions effectively.

If a client is aspirating their saliva, management would include assiduous oral care (to avoid bacteria-laden saliva entering the lungs) and positioning. Reduced spontaneous swallows may be addressed using some of the stimulation techniques described under D for direct therapy. Overproduction of saliva can be treated pharmacologically – with hyoscine, for example.

Always talk to the pharmacist if you suspect that your client's saliva production may be affected by medication.

> **✗ CLINICAL TOP TIP**
>
> Use of the term 'drooling' can be distressing for both the client and their carer, with its pejorative undertones. Clinicians should imbue the therapeutic encounter with dignity and respect by using more neutral and objective language, such as 'anterior escape of saliva'.

Y IS FOR . . .

YOGHURT

Yoghurt is often the foodstuff of choice for SLT EDS assessment involving a bolus. This is partly to do with convenience and availability, and partly to do with the fact that yoghurt is generally IDDSI Level 4 and therefore a consistency which offers reduced choking possibilities with some viscosity.

However, yoghurt can vary in consistency, from thin enough to drip from a spoon to thick and creamy (eg, Greek yoghurt) to gelatinous and set. Make sure you use one that is of a consistent texture (ie, no chunks of fruit) – managing two consistencies is always more challenging than one and chunks of fruit may also pose a choking risk.

Check that your client is not vegan or lactose intolerant – other options might include a pudding, fruit compote or thickened drink.

Some SLTs choose to begin their oral trials assessment with water. If aspiration is a possibility, water is the substance least likely to cause chest complications. However, the oral examination/CNA may suggest that control of the bolus will be problematic, in which case a more cohesive, thicker bolus (eg, yoghurt) may be preferred. Thickened water is another possibility but, as discussed earlier, most people find this highly unpalatable.

YOUR SUPPORT AND SUPERVISION

Support and supervision are important throughout your SLT career. If you graduate after 2026 in the UK, you will complete theoretical EDS learning in the classroom as well as pre-registration clinical competencies and exposure hours while out on placement (RCSLT, 2021). However, it is recognised that as you begin your career in EDS assessment and management, you will still require a high level of support. This might take the form of an in-house training package, a series of observations and joint working with a more senior colleague, or a post-registration EDS course.

Supervision on graduation is very regular and frequent (the Royal College of Speech and Language Therapists recommends every week for the first three months), and this is invaluable to help you develop as a clinician. To make the most of your supervision sessions, reflect regularly on EDS sessions with clients and bring these reflections to the session. Set the agenda for your supervision sessions so that they meet your needs. Write up notes afterwards of what you and your supervisor discussed and create an action plan. Make sure that you have the next session booked into both of your diaries.

Support can be derived from a number of sources, such as from peers (other SLTs at a similar grade to you), more experienced clinicians, your line manager and the wider MDT. You may find it easier to talk to your peers about difficult situations than to your supervisor – make sure that you keep all client details confidential in this space.

As an SLT, you will continue to receive supervision throughout your career, enabling you to continue developing even as a very experienced practitioner. Whether you are a Band 5 or a Band 8, never be afraid to ask for a second opinion when faced with a particularly thorny EDS issue.

Y CLINICAL TOP TIP

Why not start an EDS peer support group in your service or an informal lunch group?

Z IS FOR . . .

ZOOM OR EDS ASSESSMENT AND MANAGEMENT VIA TELEHEALTH

Out of adversity can come invention and creativity, and this was certainly the case during and after the COVID-19 pandemic. Eighteenth-century German philosopher Fichte (although this is often attributed to his nineteenth-century counterpart, Hegel) spoke in his dialectic of how the status quo (the thesis) can be turned upside down by a major event (the antithesis), thereby creating a synthesis. Adopting this dialectic, we might claim that out of the antithetical period of the pandemic emerged a synthesis of conventional EDS management with innovative approaches, such as the clinical use of video calls.

The reasons for choosing tele-assessment and tele-management of EDS are multifarious but may include a client's inability to travel to the clinic, time constraints or client preference. Their use may be contraindicated if the client does not have access to the required technology (through either choice or digital poverty), if they are unable to use the required technology (eg, because of cognitive impairment) or perhaps because the light source, positioning of the camera or internet provision is not optimal.

Let's consider which aspects of EDS assessment and management may be successfully carried out via Zoom. Luckily, we use our skills of observation a lot when it comes to assessing how safe the swallow is during clinical evaluation, so these observation skills can also be used via Zoom:

- orofacial musculature at rest (is there any evidence of asymmetry, weakness or spasticity?);
- observation of breathing (clavicular or diaphragmatic?);

- vocal quality;
- strength of cough;
- evidence of anterior escape of saliva, indicative of reduced buccal tension and reduced lip seal; and
- general posture.

Specific assessment strategies may also be carried out via Zoom, such as an oromotor assessment or CNA (motor components only). The clinician gives clear instructions and perhaps models specific movements for the client to copy. Mealtime observations may also be successfully carried out this way, as long as the camera allows a good view of the person eating.

Some management strategies may also be possible using this method. For example, you may be able to model head positions for your client (eg, a chin tuck) and observe them as they have a go. Similarly, you may be able to teach safer swallow manoeuvres, such as the Mendelsohn, or specific exercises, such as the Shaker. You could even consider recording these sessions, so that the client has a permanent record to which to refer. Similarly, you could go through oromotor exercises with the client in real time. The use of current safer swallowing strategies and consistencies can be observed and evaluated, as well as different ones trialled.

Discussion, advice and support can all take place virtually; as can some training of others. The use of built-in functions such as breakout rooms and the chat facility can render training via Zoom interactive, thereby ensuring deeper learning.

Innovative and useful as telehealth is proving to be for our clients with EDS needs, there are inevitably some aspects of assessment and management that do not lend themselves to this approach, including:

- anything involving the need to touch the client (eg, laryngeal palpation, testing for sensitivity, testing for strength of movement, oral care or demonstrating oral care); and
- trialling food/fluid boluses for the first time if there are any major risks of aspiration. In this instance, you will normally need the back-up of other members of the team, such as a

respiratory physiotherapist who can auscultate and check for aspiration. *In extremis*, the respiratory physiotherapist can also use suction or chest drainage.

Protocol:

- Send instructions to the client, if necessary (most people now know how Zoom works, but the client may need specific instructions regarding optimising the view through correct placement of the tablet or computer and having a good light source).
- Ensure that the client has someone with them, if necessary.

> **Z CLINICAL TOP TIP**
>
> If you are using your phone or a tablet, make sure that you hold it in landscape, not portrait, and be mindful of your background. If you often use this approach, you may want to invest in a stand to ensure optimal positioning.

APPENDIX

Indicative answers to clinical reasoning case studies (see under C)

JUDITH

Your clinical reasoning, having taken a clinical history, might include the following.

Judith had her stroke very recently (three days ago), so we might expect that the clinical picture is changing rapidly:

- The unaffected upper motor neurones (ie, those originating from the left hemisphere) which innervate the bilaterally innervated cranial nerves used in swallowing (ie, CNs V, IX and X) will take over innervation completely (although possibly asymmetrically, as discussed under C for cranial nerves).
- Oedema from damage to the cortex will start to subside, so some improvement is expected.

Damage to the right cortex around the motor strip suggests that you might see weakness of the left side of the body – including the peri-oral area (CN VII, lower branch) and the tongue (CN XII). Language difficulties are unlikely (as the stroke occurred in her non-dominant hemisphere), but she may have some motor speech difficulties (unilateral upper motor neurone dysarthria); she should be able to understand auditory commands during the CNA.

Judith was drowsy but is now alert, suggesting that she is ready for a clinical assessment.

The history of her presenting condition (transient ischaemic attacks) and past medical history of hypertension are both risk factors for stroke. There is no evidence of pre-existing pathologies which might impact EDS.

Drug history is consistent with her diagnosis of hiatus hernia; there are no side effects of this drug that should impact swallowing, but it is always worth checking with the pharmacist. The hiatus hernia is something to bear in mind when she resumes oral intake – you could seek support and advice from the dietitian.

Despite her hemiparesis, Judith is able to transfer from the bed to a chair, so it should be possible for her to be in a good, upright position for assessment.

There are no clinical signs of a current chest infection: there are no sounds on auscultation and no rise in temperature or in white blood cells, and she has excellent oxygen perfusion in her blood. This tells us two things: she is well enough to proceed with assessment and it is less likely that she has been aspirating her saliva.

She has been without food for at least three days and has no alternative means of nutrition, so she needs to be prioritised for assessment and management of her swallowing.

Table 39 shows the results of the CSE and what these might tell us.

- Oral preparatory stage: Reduced ability to manipulate, control and contain the bolus.
- Oral stage: Reduced ability to move the bolus anterior-posteriorly; reduced intraoral pressure.
- Pharyngeal stage: No clinical evidence of delayed swallow reflex; good cough.

In terms of diagnosis, we know that Judith's EDS needs came about as a result of a stroke (neurogenic); that the oral preparatory, oral and (possibly) pharyngeal stages are affected (oropharyngeal); and that she is showing some signs of aspiration and/or laryngeal penetration on small amounts of a thin (IDDSI Level 0) bolus, but not on IDDSI Levels 1, 2 and 4. We might give a tentative diagnosis at this stage such as this:

> Judith presents with moderate neurogenic oropharyngeal dysphagia, characterised by reduced rate, range and strength of tongue and lip movement on the left.

Table 39 Results of Judith's clinical swallow examination and what these might tell us

Clinical assessment with rationale	Findings	What this means
CNA Rationale: Client is alert and talking – unlikely to have difficulties obeying commands.	V: Good mouth opening, slightly reduced strength left side of jaw.	Mouth-opening adequate for oral trials, although anterior escape may be an issue. Mastication may be mildly affected.
	VII: Reduced range and strength of movement of lips on left, air/saliva escape left side.	May have difficulties keeping the bolus in the oral cavity and saliva may escape anteriorly. Intra-oral pressure may be reduced, making anterior-posterior movement of the bolus more difficult.
	X: Strong volitional cough, voicing clear, soft palate symmetrical on /a/.	Suggests good airway protection. Velar movement suggests good velopharyngeal closure which helps with intra-oral pressure. Nasal regurgitation unlikely to be an issue.
	XII: Reduced range of movement and reduced strength left side of tongue, reduced rate of lateral movement, tongue deviates to left on protrusion.	Reduction in rate, range and strength of movement of the tongue will affect manipulation of the bolus, anterior-posterior propulsion and ability to retrieve bolus from the lateral sulci.
Laryngeal palpation Rationale: Client should understand what you are doing and why.	Good forward and upward movement of the larynx felt. Prompt dry swallow.	Suggestive of no delay in swallow trigger, with adequate airway protection and cricopharyngeal opening.

(Continued)

Table 39 (Continued)

Clinical assessment with rationale	Findings	What this means
Oral trials Rationale: Client is alert and has demonstrated ability to protect airway. She is able to sit upright. No clinical signs of current chest infection. Oral movements suggest possible oral preparatory and oral stage difficulties.	Trial 1 (water from spoon): Anterior escape of water (L), prompt swallow, throat-clear post-swallow.	Reduced lip seal left side, leading to reduced ability to contain the bolus in the oral cavity. Throat-clear suggestive of laryngeal penetration by the bolus with attempt to clear.
	Trial 2 (water from cup): Anterior escape of water, prompt swallow, cough post-swallow.	Reduced lip seal left side, leading to reduced ability to contain the bolus in the oral cavity. Cough suggestive of frank laryngeal penetration or aspiration by the bolus with attempt to clear.
	Trial 3 (IDDSI Level 2 – thickened squash from cup): No anterior escape of the bolus, prompt swallow elicited. No cough. Voice clear post-swallow.	Bolus contained within oral cavity and no clinical signs of aspiration.
	Trial 4 (IDDSI Level 1): As above.	
	Trial 5 (IDDSI Level 4 – yoghurt): No anterior escape of bolus, prompt swallow elicited. Voice clear post-swallow. No cough.	Bolus contained within oral cavity and no clinical signs of aspiration.
	Trial 6 (yoghurt): As above.	

Your next steps might include the following:

- Recommend small amounts of IDDSI Level 4 food intake (5–10 teaspoons yoghurt, twice a day) and IDDSI Level 1 fluids (100 ml via cup, twice a day, small sips) over the next day. Must be seated upright.
- Nursing staff to observe any clinical signs of aspiration and monitor chest status.
- SLT review in 1/7.

Did you think about any other assessment techniques that you might use? For example, you might want to use pulse oximetry and/or cervical auscultation during the oral trials. I don't think I would refer her to videofluoroscopy or FEES at this stage because her clinical picture is probably changing.

PRAKASH

Your clinical reasoning, having taken a clinical history, may include the following.

The site of Prakash's lesion (pons and medulla) suggests that there could be profound difficulties with both speech and swallowing, because CNs V and VII originate in the pons and CNs IX, X and XII in the medulla. The cranial nerves synapse in the brainstem with the upper motor neurones, so both upper motor neurone (spastic) and lower motor neurone (flaccid) signs may be in evidence.

Past medical history shows that his chest status may already be compromised by asthma. Hypertension and non-insulin dependent diabetes mellitus are both risk factors for stroke. Depression is common after stroke – Prakash has a pre-existing diagnosis of depression, so this may be exacerbated.

Drug history includes medications that can cause xerostomia (fluoxetine and salbutamol) and a dry cough (lisinopril).

Prakash's arousal level is high enough for a CSE (we normally need a GCS of at least 11/15 before attempting a CSE). He is likely to understand the reason for the assessment and any auditory commands, as the lesion has affected his brainstem and not the cortex, which houses all his thinking and language skills.

APPENDIX 165

Table 40 Questions asked by the SLT during case history taking, Meera and Prakash's responses and how these help with clinical decision-making

SLT	Meera	Prakash	What does this tell us?
'Can you tell me a bit about what has happened to you?'	Been in hospital for 14 days – admitted by ambulance after collapsing at home. Doctors have informed them that Prakash has had a brainstem stroke.		Prakash and Meera know what the diagnosis is.
'Did you have any difficulties with eating and drinking prior to this?'	No – nothing.	Looks down for no.	Prakash had no pre-existing difficulties with EDS – this gives us a baseline.
'Do you have any pain when you swallow?'		Looks down for no.	Odynophagia is rare in neurogenic dysphagia – this confirms that Prakash is not experiencing pain on swallowing.
'Have you had any chest problems since you came into hospital?'	Explains that he had a short course of antibiotics shortly after admission but these have now stopped and so has the coughing.	Looks up for yes.	This is an indication that Prakash might have aspirated (saliva/vomitus?) when he was first admitted, which caused a chest infection.
'Did you have problems with breathing or coughing before you came into hospital?'		Prakash indicates yes and spells out 'inhaler' on E-Tran frame.	This confirms our knowledge about Prakash's asthma.

(*Continued*)

Table 40 (Continued)

SLT	Meera	Prakash	What does this tell us?
'Is there anything you want to ask me?'	Meera explains that they do not eat meat, eggs or fish for religious reasons.	Indicates 'no meat' using the E-Tran frame. Spells out 'food when'.	This helps us to understand Prakash's religious needs. The final question addresses prognosis and is always a difficult one for the clinician. Although the prognosis looks bleak because of the size and location of the lesion, it is too early on in the rehabilitation phase to be definitive.

Table 41 The rationale for and results of Prakash's CSE and what these might tell us

Clinical assessment component and rationale	Result	What this tells us
Oral hygiene exam. Rationale: Prakash is NBM – if he is aspirating, it is important that saliva is kept as clean as possible. Not eating and drinking means that oral hygiene may be compromised.	Dry saliva around lips and adhering to hard palate. White patches on tongue.	Dried saliva may indicate open mouth posture and mouth-breathing. Oral care may not be optimal. White patches are an indication of candida albicans (thrush).
CNA. Rationale: Prakash is alert enough and has the cognition/language skills to participate.	V: Reduced mouth-opening. Weak movement against resistance. Poor lateral jaw movement. Intra-oral and peri-oral sensation not assessed. VII: Lips symmetrical at rest, low tone. Approximate /i/ and /u/ but slow. Anterior escape of saliva in evidence. Air escape noted via lips when client asked to puff up cheeks. X: Soft palate looks symmetrical at rest – client able to produce weak /a/. Some nasal escape noted when client asked to puff up cheeks.	Difficulty introducing bolus. Reduced mouth closure. Reduced mastication. Reduced ability to shape lips around spoon/cup. Reduced lip seal resulting in reduced intraoral pressure and anterior escape of saliva/food/drink. Some movement of velum but velopharyngeal closure incomplete – possible nasal regurgitation and effect on intraoral pressure.

(*Continued*)

Table 41 (Continued)

Clinical assessment component and rationale	Result	What this tells us
	Able to cough to command – reduced strength.	Some laryngeal function but reduced strength.
	XII: Tongue symmetrical and flaccid at rest. Fasciculations noted. Reduced ability to protrude tongue and move tongue laterally. Unable to push tongue into cheek, unable to lick lips.	Symmetry suggests bilateral weakness. Fasciculations suggest lower motor neurone (flaccid) signs. Reduced ability to manipulate and control the bolus, retrieve parts of the bolus from the sulci and anterior-posterior propulsion of the bolus.
Laryngeal palpation Rationale: Prakash will be able to understand the need for and consent to laryngeal palpation.	Reduced hyolaryngeal excursion with suspected prolonged oral-prep and oral stages.	Possible delay in swallow trigger. Compromised airway protection. Reduced opening of cricopharyngeal sphincter.

(*Continued*)

Table 41 (Continued)

Clinical assessment component and rationale	Result	What this tells us
Oral trials Rationale: Prakash is alert and can be seated in an upright position, in either a chair or a profiling bed. CNA has identified that oral control will be problematic, so thin consistencies not trialled.	1st bolus: 1 x teaspoon smooth yoghurt (IDDSI Level 4). Opened mouth slightly to approach of spoon. Prolonged oral preparatory stage with ++ tongue-pumping and some anterior escape. Swallow elicited – cough post-swallow. No oral residue noted but difficult to see into mouth because of reduced mouth-opening. 2nd bolus: 1 x teaspoon smooth yoghurt (IDDSI Level 4). Opened mouth slightly to approach of spoon. Prolonged oral preparatory stage with ++ tongue-pumping and some anterior escape. Swallow elicited – no cough post-swallow. No oral residue noted but difficult to see into mouth because of reduced mouth-opening. Sats dropped from 98% to 94% after swallow trials.	Reduced control of the bolus in oral cavity and ability to transfer the bolus from front to back of mouth. Possible delay in swallow trigger. Cough post-swallow indicates laryngeal penetration or aspiration. Drop in oxygen saturations may indicate aspiration.

He is vocalising, which indicates some laryngeal involvement, but he is not producing any intelligible speech sounds, which may indicate very severe dysarthria or anarthria.

The oral preparatory stage will be affected because Prakash is unable to move his arms and therefore will be unable to bring food and drink to his mouth. You will need to make sure that he has been transferred to a chair or that he is seated upright in a profiling bed before you can proceed with the CSE.

Although Prakash is NBM, he does have an alternative means of deriving hydration and nutrition (NGT), so although his dysphagia is more severe, he is less of a priority for assessment than Judith.

His chest status is good, with no signs of infection (ie, no crepitations heard and temperature and white cell count normal). Oxygen saturations are slightly down, but this may be because of his asthma.

The case history and CSE results and what these may tell us are outlined in the tables above.

Your diagnosis might look something like this:

> Prakash presents with severe neurogenic oropharyngeal dysphagia, characterised by severely reduced rate, range and strength of oral movements, a possible delay in the swallow reflex and reduced ability to protect the airway. He is currently unsafe on all oral intake.

You next steps might include the following:

- Talking to Prakash and Meera about your findings, especially in view of Prakash's question about prognosis. How much detail people want will differ from person to person. Although it is probable that Prakash will be left with significant EDS needs, we cannot know at this stage exactly what these will be – it is important to be realistic and honest with clients and carers, but also not to deprive them of hope.
- Watchful waiting – reviewing Prakash's swallow clinically in a week's time to check for any spontaneous progress.

- Implementing oromotor exercises to try to increase the rate, range and strength of the lip and tongue muscles.
- Referral to the medical team for treatment of thrush and to the nursing team for assiduous oral care.
- Videofluoroscopy might be merited even at this early stage in Prakash's rehabilitation. This would give us a detailed baseline of his swallowing skills and would confirm the delay in swallow trigger and aspiration.

TOMMY

Tommy may not have had any EDS symptoms related to his tumour, but he is beginning to experience adverse side effects from the curative radiotherapy. Although targeted to the tumour, healthy tissue will also be affected.

He was probably eating a full oral diet prior to commencement of treatment, but with your help he may now have to decide on some modifications to make eating and drinking safe and more pleasurable (see table 42).

Your diagnosis might be:

> Tommy presents with moderate iatrogenic dysphagia related to radiotherapy treatment for a parotid salivary gland tumour, characterised by acute mucositis and trismus, chronic fibrosis and reduction in saliva production, resulting in odynophagia and reduced enjoyment of eating and drinking.

DERVLA

Dervla has a neurodegenerative diagnosis, so we know that the trajectory of her EDS difficulties is one of decline. The first neurological signs experienced by someone with motor neurone disease may well be changes to their swallowing and the time from diagnosis to death is quite short (usually between two and five years). The aim of your SLT intervention is therefore to help Dervla eat and drink as safely and as comfortably as possible for as long as possible.

Table 42 Symptoms, cause and possible management strategies for EDS issues associated with radiotherapy for head and neck cancer

Symptom	Cause	Possible management strategy
Reduced saliva	Radiation damage to the parotid salivary gland (and possibly others)	Recommend sips of fluid between mouthfuls of food. Sucking ice chips. Artificial saliva products. This damage is likely to be permanent, so long-term acceptable strategies need to be found.
Pain on swallowing	Mucositis	Discuss different textures and tastes with Tommy and draw up menus in consultation with the dietitian. Reassure Tommy that, although mucositis will get worse as treatment continues (and may remain several weeks after treatment), it should resolve over time.
Reduced mouth-opening	Trismus	Recommend spoon with shallow bowl. Implementation of mouth-opening exercises, such as use of TheraBite (Atos Medical), or stacks of wooden tongue depressors. This intervention should be started as soon as possible for best results.
Effortful swallowing	Fibrosis	Stiffening of structures can be a permanent difficulty after radiotherapy. Gentle exercises to keep the jaw, tongue and lips mobile may be useful.
Loss of enjoyment of eating and drinking	Reduced saliva production, odynophagia, mucositis, fibrosis and damaged taste receptors may all be impacting enjoyment of eating and drinking.	Discuss diet and menus with Tommy and the dietitian.
Weight loss	Reduced intake	Discussion with dietitian about food choices and possible supplements. Enteral feeding may need to be considered, to augment or replace oral intake during treatment.

Her current presentation suggests that she is already experiencing changes to swallow physiology – for example, her tongue movements have slowed (affecting control and manipulation of the bolus and anterior-posterior movement), and the bolus is entering into the pharynx before the swallow is triggered, meaning that the airway is open and unprotected while there is material in the pharynx. She is coughing on some consistencies, indicative of laryngeal penetration, if not aspiration. She has a reduced ability to protect her airway because her cough reflex is weak. However, despite all this, she has not had any chest infections, which may mean that she is tolerating some aspiration or that her weak cough is still managing to eject any material from the laryngeal vestibule.

The diagnosis we supply in a report might look like this:

> Dervla presents with moderate neurogenic oropharyngeal dysphagia, characterised by slow rate of tongue movements, a delay in the swallow reflex and possible laryngeal penetration or aspiration.

Because the progression of the disease is quick, you will need to review and support Dervla regularly, being reactive to any changes in her EDS presentation. With Dervla, you could discuss avoiding particularly problematic food, head and body positioning and swallow manoeuvres. She may even be amenable to texture modification.

At this relatively early stage of the disease, it is worth talking about future interventions with Dervla while she has functional speech. Discuss her feelings about texture modification and enteral feeding. Explain fully and candidly what aspiration is and what the consequences might be. Explain what a PEG is – you might want to do this session with the dietitian.

Dervla's opinions about when (if ever) to go down the enteral feeding route are paramount. She may decide that she never wants enteral feeding and to continue to eat and drink orally until she dies. She will need to discuss an advance directive with her GP. These sorts of decisions need constant reviewing and updating.

Your relationship with Dervla as she starts to experience these changes to her swallowing is absolutely key. It is vital that you are honest with her, so that trust ensues. Your support and advice will be invaluable to Dervla and those around her as she faces this horrible disease.

Don't forget to seek your own support and supervision as you navigate Dervla's swallowing journey.

REFERENCES

Adams, V., Mathisen, B., Baines, S., Lazarus, C., and Callister, R. (2013) A Systematic Review and Meta-analysis of Measurements of Tongue and Hand Strength and Endurance Using the Iowa Oral Performance Instrument (IOPI). *Dysphagia* 28, 350–369 (2013). https://doi.org/10.1007/s00455-013-9451-3

Alamer, A., Melese, H., and Nigussie, F. (2020). Effectiveness of Neuromuscular Electrical Stimulation on Post-Stroke Dysphagia: A Systematic Review of Randomized Controlled Trials. *Clinical Interventions in Aging*, 15, 1521–1531. https://doi.org/10.2147/CIA.S262596

Amathieu, R., Sauvat, S., Reynaud, P., Slavov, V., Luis, D., Dinca, A., and Dhonneur, G. (2012) Influence of the Cuff Pressure on the Swallowing Reflex in Tracheostomized Intensive Care Unit Patients. *British Journal of Anaesthesia*, 109(4), 578–583.

Archer, S.K., Smith, C.H., and Newham, D.J. (2021) Surface Electromyographic Biofeedback and the Effortful Swallow Exercise for Stroke-Related Dysphagia and in Healthy Ageing. *Dysphagia* 36, 281–292 (2021). https://doi.org/10.1007/s00455-020-10129-8

Baker, C., Worrall, L., Rose, M., and Ryan, B. (2020) 'It Was Really Dark': The Experiences and Preferences of People with Aphasia to Manage Mood Changes and Depression. *Aphasiology*, 34(1), 19–46.

Beauchamp, T. L. and Childress, J. F. (1979) *Principles of Biomedical Ethics*. Oxford University Press.

Béchet, S., Hill, F., Gilheaney, O., and Walshe, M. (2016) Diagnostic Accuracy of the Modified Evan's Blue Dye Test in Detecting Aspiration in Patients with Tracheostomy: A Systematic Review of the Evidence. *Dysphagia* 31(6), 721–729.

Brates, D., Molfenter, S. M. and Thibeault, S.L. (2019) Assessing Hyolaryngeal Excursion: Comparing Quantitative Methods to Palpation at the Bedside and Visualization During Videofluoroscopy. *Dysphagia*, 34, 298–307.

Brooke, J. and Ojo, O. (2015) Enteral Nutrition in Dementia: A Systematic Review. *Nutrients*, 7, 2456–2468.

Brooks, M., McLaughlin, E., and Shields, N. (2017) Expiratory Muscle Strength Training Improves Swallowing and Respiratory Outcomes in People with Dysphagia: A Systematic Review. *International Journal of Speech-Language Pathology*, 21(1), 89–100. https://doi.org/10.1080/17549507.2017.1387285

Cambridge Dictionary CULTURE | English meaning - Cambridge Dictionary, https://dictionary.cambridge.org/dictionary/english/culture (accessed 1 September 2024).

Crary, M.A., Mann, G.D., and Groher, M.E. (2005) Initial Psychometric Assessment of a Functional Oral Intake Scale for Dysphagia in Stroke Patients. *Archives of Physical Medicine and Rehabilitation* 86(8), 1516–1520.

Dietrich, T., Webb, I., Stenhouse, L., Pattni, A., Ready, D., Wanyonyi, K.L., White, S., and Gallagher, J.E. (2017) Evidence Summary: The Relationship Between Oral and Cardiovascular Disease. *British Dental Journal*, 222, 381–385. https://doi.org/10.1038/sj.bdj.2017.224

Enderby, P. and John, A. (2015) *Therapy Outcome Measures for Rehabilitation Professionals (3rd edition)*. J and R Press.

Enderby, P. and John, A. (2025) Therapy Outcome Measure: Scales and resources for nutrition, eating, drinking and swallowing. J and R Press

Engel, G.L. (1977) The Need for a New Medical Model: A Challenge for Biomedicine. *Science* 196(4286), 129–136.

Finucane, T.E., Christmas, C., and Travis, K. (1999) Tube Feeding in Patients with Advanced Dementia: A Review of the Evidence. *Journal of the American Medical Association*, 1999, 282, 1365–1370.

Frank, A.W. (2013) *The Wounded Storyteller: Body, Illness and Ethics* (second edition). University of Chicago Press

Fujiu, M. and Logemann, J-L. (1996) Effect of a Tongue-Holding Maneuver on Posterior Pharyngeal Wall Movement During Deglutition. *American Journal of Speech-Language Pathology*, 5(1), 23–30.

Gilmore, R., Aram, J., Powell, J., and Greenwood, R. (2003) Treatment of Oro-Facial Hypersensitivity Following Brain Injury. *Brain Injury*, 17(4), 347–354. https://doi.org/10.1080/0269905031000070233

Gillman, A., Winkler, R., and Taylor, N. (2017) Implementing the Free Water Protocol Does Not Result in Aspiration Pneumonia in Carefully Selected Patients with Dysphagia: A Systematic Review. *Dysphagia*, 32, 345–361.

Gross, R., Mahlmann, J., and Grayhack, J. (2003) Physiologic Effects of Open and Closed Tracheostomy Tubes on the Pharyngeal Swallow. *Annals of Otology, Rhinology & Laryngology*, 112(2), 143–152.

Hägg, M. and Tibbling, L. (2016) Effect of IQoro® Training on Impaired Postural Control and Oropharyngeal Motor Function in Patients with Dysphagia after Stroke. *Acta Oto-Laryngologica*, 136(7), 742–748.

Hansen, T., Beck, A M., Kjaersgaard, A., and Poulsen, I. (2022) Second Update of a Systematic Review and Evidence-Based Recommendations on Texture Modified Foods and Thickened Liquids for Adults (Above 17 Years) with Oropharyngeal Dysphagia. *Clinical Nutrition ESPEN*, 49, June.

Hansjee, D. (2018) Risk Feeding: From Protocol to Model of Care. *Royal College of Speech & Language Therapists Bulletin*, 789.

Hansjee, D., Burch, N., Campbell, L., Crawford, H., Crowder, R., Garrett, D., Harp, K., Howells, G., Morris, J., Pasco, K., Rochford, A., Ruck Keene, A., Slater, T., Smith, A., Smithard, D. and Stanier, J. (2021) Eating and drinking with acknowledged risks: Multidisciplinary team guidance for the shared decision-making process (adults). RCSLT

Hepper, E. C., Wilson, J., Drinnan, M., and Patterson, J. M. (2024) Psychosocial Impacts of Being Nil-By-Mouth as an Adult: A Scoping Review. *Journal of Advanced Nursing*, 80, 3499–3515.

Hersh, D., Worrall, L., Howe, T., Sherratt, S., and Davidson, B. (2012) SMARTER Goal Setting in Aphasia Rehabilitation. *Aphasiology*, 26(1).

Hughes, T.A. and Wiles, C.M. (1996) Clinical Measurement of Swallowing in Health and in Neurogenic Dysphagia. *QJM*, 89, 109–16.

Hwang, N-K., Kim, H-H., Shim, J-M., and Park, J-S. (2019) Tongue Stretching Exercises Improve Tongue Motility and Oromotor Function in Patients with Dysphagia After Stroke: A Preliminary Randomized Controlled Trial. *Archives of Oral Biology*, 108.

Jaghbeer, M., Sutt, A-L., and Bergström, L. (2023) Dysphagia Management and Cervical Auscultation: Reliability and Validity Against FEES. *Dysphagia*, 38, 305–314.

Kang, J. Y., Choi, K. H., Yun, G J., Kim, M. Y., and Ryu, J. S. (2012) Does Removal of Tracheostomy Affect Dysphagia? A Kinematic Analysis. *Dysphagia*, 27, 498–503.

Kawakami, M., Simeoni, S., Tremblay, S., Hannah, R., Fujiwara, T., and Rothwell, J.C. (2019) Changes in the Excitability of Corticobulbar Projections Due to Intraoral Cooling with Ice. *Dysphagia*, 34, 708–712.

Kitamura, K., Watanabe, T., Yamamoto, M, Ishikawa, N., Kasahara, N., Abe, S., and Yamamoto, H. (2022) A Newly Discovered Tendon Between the Genioglossus Muscle and Epiglottic Cartilage Identified by Histological Observation of the Pre-Epiglottic Space. *Dysphagia*, 38, 315–329.

Langmore, S. and Pisegna, J. (2015) Efficacy of Exercises to Rehabilitate Dysphagia: A Critique of the Literature. *International Journal of Speech-Language Pathology*, 17(3), 222–229.

Langmore, S., Terpenning, M.S., Schork, A., Chen, Y., Murray, J. T., Lopatin, D., and Loesche, W. J. (1998) Predictors of Aspiration Pneumonia: How Important Is Dysphagia? *Dysphagia*, 13, 69–81.

Leadership Alliance for the Care of Dying People (2014) *One Chance to Get it Right.* https://assets.publishing.service.gov.uk/media/5a7e301ced915d74e33f09ee/One_chance_to_get_it_right.pdf (accessed 24 October 2024).

Logemann, J. A. (1996) *Evaluation and Treatment of Swallowing Disorders.* Pro-ed.

MacKenzie, S. (2017) *Mosaics, Ambiguity and Quest: Constructing Stories of Spirituality with People with Expressive Aphasia.* PhD Thesis Canterbury Christ Church University Faculty of Health and Wellbeing. https://repository.canterbury.ac.uk/item/8862z/mosaics-ambiguity-and-quest-constructing-stories-of-spirituality-with-people-with-expressive-aphasia (accessed 7 September 2024).

MacKenzie, S. (2024) *Working with Adults with Eating, Drinking and Swallowing Needs: A Holistic Approach.* Routledge.

MacKenzie, S. and Mumby, K. (eds) (2022) *Perspectives on Spirituality in Speech and Language Therapy.* J and R Press.

Mathisen, B., Carey, L. B., Carey-Sargeant, C. L., Webb, G., Millar, C., and Krikheli, L. (2015) Religion, Spirituality and Speech-Language Pathology: A Viewpoint for Ensuring Patient-Centred Holistic Care. *Journal of Religion and Health*, 54, 2309–2323.

Mental Capacity Act 2005, c 9. https://www.legislation.gov.uk/ukpga/2005/9/contents/enacted (accessed 30 January 2025).

Mepani, R., Antonik, S., Massey, B., Kern, M., Logemann, J., Pauloski, B., Rademaker, A., Easterling, C., and Shaker, R. (2009) Augmentation of Deglutitive Thyrohyoid Muscle Shortening by the Shaker Exercise. *Dysphagia*, 24(1), 26–31.

Miles, A., Jardine, M., Johnston, F., de Lisle, M., Friary, P., and Allen, J. (2017) Effect of Lee Silverman Voice Treatment (LSVT LOUD®) on Swallowing and Cough in Parkinson's Disease: A Pilot Study. *Journal of the Neurological Sciences*, 383, 180–187.

MBSImP Modified Barium Swallow Impairment Profile (northern speech.com). https://www.northernspeech.com/mbsimp/ (accessed 20 August 2024).

Nozaki, S., Fujiu-Kurachi, M., Tanimura, T., Ishizuka, K., Miyata, E., Sugishita, S., Imai, T., Nishiguchi, M., Furuta, M., and Yorifuji, S. (2021) Effects of Lee Silverman Voice Treatment (LSVT LOUD) on Swallowing in Patients with Progressive Supranuclear Palsy: A Pilot Study. *Progress in Rehabilitation Medicine*, 6.

Panther, K. (2005) The Frazier Free Water Protocol. *Perspectives on Swallowing and Swallowing Disorders – ASHA*, March.

Papadopoulou, S., Exarchakos, G., Beris, A., and Ploumis, A. (2013) Dysphagia Associated with Cervical Spine and Postural Disorders. *Dysphagia*, 28, 469–480.

Park, M. K. and Lee, S. J. (2018) Changes in Swallowing and Cough Functions Among Stroke Patients Before and After Tracheostomy Decannulation. *Dysphagia*, 33, 857–865.

Peña-Chávez, R. E., Schaen-Heacock, N. E., Hitchcock, M. E., Kurosu, A., Suzuki, R., Hartel, R., Ciucci, M., and Rogus-Pulia, N. (2023) Effects of Food and Liquid Properties on Swallowing Physiology and Function in Adults. *Dysphagia*, 38, 785–817. https://doi.org/10.1007/s00455-022-10525-2

Regan, J., (2020) Impact of Sensory Stimulation on Pharyngo-Esophageal Swallowing Biomechanics in Adults with Dysphagia: A High-Resolution Manometry Study. *Dysphagia*, 35(5), 825–833.

Roa Pauloski, B., Logemann, J. A., Rademaker, A. W., Lundy, D., Sullivan, P. A., Newman, L. A., Lazarus, C., and Bacon, M. (2013) Effects of Enhanced Bolus Flavors on Oropharyngeal Swallow in Patients Treated for Head and Neck Cancer. *Head & Neck*, 35(8), 1124–1131.

Rogers, C. (1951) *Client-Centered Therapy*. Constable.

Rosenbek, J. C., Robbins, J. A., Roecker, E. B., Coyle, J. L., and Wood, J. L. (1996) A Penetration-Aspiration Scale. *Dysphagia*, 11(2), 93–98.

Royal College of Speech and Language Therapists (2021) *RCSLT Competencies in Eating, Drinking, and Swallowing for the Pre-Registration Education and Training of Speech and Language Therapists*. https://www.rcslt.org/wp-content/uploads/2021/11/RCSLT-Competencies-in-EDS-for-pre-registration-education-and-training-of-SLTs_OCT-2021.pdf (accessed 12 January 2025).

Sdravou, K., Walshe, M., and Dagdilelis, L. (2012) Effects of Carbonated Liquids on Oropharyngeal Swallowing Measures in People with Neurogenic Dysphagia. *Dysphagia*, 27, 240–250.

Shaker, R., Kern, M., Bardan, E., Taylor, A., Stewart, E. T., Hoffmann, R. G, Arndorfer, C., Hofmann, C., and Bonnevier, J. (1997) Augmentation of Deglutitive Upper Esophageal Sphincter Opening in the Elderly by Exercise. *American Journal of Physiology.*, 272 (6 Pt 1), 1518–1522.

Smithard, D. G., Swaine, I., Ayis, S., Gambaruto, A., Stone-Ghariani, A., Hansjee, D. Kulnik, S. T., Kyberd, P., Lloyd-Dehler, E., and Oliff, W. (2022) Chin Tuck against Resistance Exercise with Feedback to Improve Swallowing, Eating and Drinking in Frail Older People Admitted to Hospital with Pneumonia: Protocol for a Feasibility Randomised Controlled Study. *Pilot and Feasibility Studies* 8(105).

Sulmasy, D. P. (2002) A Biopsychosocial-Spiritual Model for the Care of Patients at the End of Life. *The Gerontologist*, 42(3), 24–33.

Swain, J., French, S., Barnes, C., and Thomas, C. (2013) *Disabling Barriers – Enabling Environments*. Sage.

Swan, K., Speyer, R., Heijnen, B. J., Wagg, B., and Cordier, R. (2015) Living with Oropharyngeal Dysphagia: Effects of Bolus Modification on Health-Related Quality of Life—A Systematic Review. *Quality of Life Research*, 24, 2447–2456.

Troche, M. S., Okun, M. S., Rosenbek, J. C., Musson, N., Fernandez, H. H., Rodriguez, R., Romrell, J., Pitts, T., Wheeler-Hegland, K. M. and Sapienza, C. M. (2010) Aspiration and Swallowing in Parkinson Disease and Rehabilitation With EMST: A Randomized Trial. *Neurology,* Nov. https://doi.org/10.1212/WNL.0b013e3181fef115

Tsikoudas, A., Barnes, M., and White, P. (2011) The Impact of Tracheostomy on the Nose. *European Archives of Oto-Rhino-Laryngology*, 268(7), 1005–1008.

Van Manen, M. (2016) *Phenomenology of Practice*. Routledge.

World Health Organization (2001) *International Classification of Disability, Functioning and Health.*

Yoon, W. L., Khoo, J. K. P. and Rickard Liow, S. J. (2014) Chin Tuck Against Resistance (CTAR): New Method for Enhancing Suprahyoid Muscle Activity Using a Shaker-Type Exercise. *Dysphagia*, 29, 243–248.

INDEX

A
acqreruired conditions, 70
acquired dysphagia, 69–70
adaptive cutlery, usage, 71
advance directive
 creation, 57
 usage, 70
aetiology
 cause, understanding, 1
 example, 15
afferent pathways (sensory pathways), importance, 105
ageing, 8
age-related muscle weakness (sarcopenia), 114
air flows, 130–131
airway
 larynx protection, 95
 obstruction, cause, 115
 protection, reduction, 115
amylase, impact, 151
anastomosis (tissue, joining), 6
anatomical arrangement, 6
anatomical structures, **9–10**
anatomy, 8–15
 alteration, 115
 musculature, 11–12
 structures, 9–11
anatomy, alteration, 1
 surgery, usage, 2, 5
anoxic brain injury, 16, 57
anterior hyolaryngeal excursion, increase, 99–100
anterior-posterior movement, 173

anterior-posterior transference, aiding, 13
anxiety, occurrence, 70
appetite, suppression, 54
arousal level, 164
articulators, 131
arytenoid cartilages, 96
arytenoids, observation, 61
aspirated material, hearing, 15
aspirating material, risk, 105
aspiration, 15–17
 clinical signs, 17
 diagnosis, 17
 impossibility, 6
 likelihood, assessment, 31
 overt aspiration, visualisation, 62
 pneumonia, 17, 110
 pneumonia, triggering, 148
 post-swallow risk, 94
 prevention, 133
 result, 115
 signs, 65
 silent aspiration, 17
aspiration risk, 16, 114, 116, 129
 avoidance, 124
 minimisation, 32
 severity
atherosclerotic vascular/ cardiovascular disease, problem, 110
autonomic nervous system, innervation, 151–152
axons, sensory information (travel), 12

B

baby foods, avoidance, 37
barium sulphate, usage, 141
bedside assessment, 31
behavioural pathology, 114
beneficence, 124
bilateral innervation, 106
bilaterality, unevenness, 38
biofeedback, supply, 144
biological/psychological/social/
    spiritual/cultural aspects,
    interaction, *69*
biopsychosocial model, 69
biopsychosocial-spiritual model,
    usage, 63, 69
Bland, Tony (anoxic brain
    injury), 57
blood flow, reduction, 46
blood glucose levels, dietitian
    monitoring, 85–86
blood vessels, inflammation, 110
body
    paralysis (hemiplegia), 112
    position, changes, 113
    posture, 75
    structure, targeting, 67
    weakness (hemiparesis), 112
body mass index (BMI), dietitian
    monitoring, 85–86
bolus, 18–19
    anterior-posterior
        transference, 13
    fluid boluses, thickening, 19
    formation, 46
        difficulty, 18–19
        saliva viscosity, changes, 19
    manipulation, 18, 173
    movement, duration, 14
    pathway, 97, 140
    second clearing swallow, 124
    transfer, 21
    trials, repetitions, 146
bony mandible, forefinger
    (usage), 98
bony protrusions (spurs), 114

brain
    injury, impact, 103
    synapse (motor/sensory
        cortices), neurones
        (conveyance), 37–38
brainstem
    cranial nerves, origination, 38
    functioning, 57
    synapsing, 106
brainstem stroke, **3**
    occurrence, 26
breathing
    cessation, apnoea, 14
    normality, 131
    observation, 158
    pattern, 31
breath support, reduction, 30
buccal musculature, weakening,
    122
buccal tension, 13, 19
    lip seal, combination, 152
buccal tone, reduction, 122
buccinator, 19

C

cancer, radiotherapy (usage), 30
candida albicans, build-up, 6
canines, cutting ability, 46
cardiorespiratory system,
    assessment/management, 88
carers
    case history, 118–120
    loss, sense, 70
    meaning, 84
    questions, **120**
cartilage, elasticity, 57
case history, 118, **118–119**
    information-gathering, 63
    questions, **28**
case history-taking, 74
    problems, 135
    SLT questions, **165–166**
ceremonies, impact, 84–85
cervical auscultation, 16, 21
    usage, 21–22

cervical spine, rigidity, 115
chaos, 76
　narrative, 77
chaplain
　liaison, 72
　role, 84–85
chest complications, 155
chest infections
　absence, 30
　development, 17
chest signs, 115
chest status, 164
　monitoring, 129
chest X-rays, interpretation/ reading, 88, 89
Cheyne-Stokes breathing, 54
chin tuck, compensatory strategies, 7
chin tuck against resistance (CTAR), 50
choking, 15–17
　hazard, 54–55, 129
　occurrence/sequelae, 16
　sensation, 138
chronic obstructive pulmonary disease (COPD), 17, 148
clavicular breathing, 158
cleft uvula, presence, 138
client
　biofeedback, supply, 144
　care, training, 86
　competence, acknowledgement, 75–76
　details, 126
　EDS needs, mapping, **79**
　empowerment, 79
　focus, 85
　functioning, details, 84
　health status, 84
　intervention, outcome (measurement), 66
　low arousal level, 31
　narrative, understanding, 78
　neurological impairment, 100
　observation, 31
　positioning, 87
　preference, 157
　pre-treatment/post-treatment status, 66
　psychological/social/spiritual/ religious/cultural needs, support, 74
　questions, 118–120
　radiotherapy treatment, 90
　trauma, 130
　VF referral, reason, 143–144
clinical assessment, readiness, 160
clinical decision-making process, 8
clinical EDS assessment, 101
clinical exam, 31
clinical history, 22, 118
　completion, 27
　information-gathering, 63
clinical reasoning, 22, 25–28
　case studies, indicative answers, 160
clinical scenarios, indicative answers, 31
clinical swallow examination (CSE), 16, 17, 21, 31–32, 80
　bolus location uncertainty, 60
　elements, 31, 99
　rationale/results, **167–169**
　results, **26**, 28, **162–163**
　usage, 134
clinician-knows-best attitude, 74–75
cognition, patient requirement, 141
cognitive behavioural therapy, 89
cognitive difficulties, 119
collaborative goal-setting, 68
　compromise, 63–64
collaborative, specific, measurable, appropriate/ achievable, realistic/ relevant, and timebound (C-SMART), 64

compensatory strategies, 7, 32–37
congruence, tenets, 121
connective tissue, presence (uvula), 138
constipation
  occurrence, barium ingestion (impact), 144
  origin, 61
continuing professional development (CPD)
  opportunities, 93
  role, 92–93
contralateral, term (reference), 106
contrast material, mixing, 91
conversation, termination, 27
corniculate cartilages, 96
cortex, unilateral damage, 19
cough
  post-swallow, 29
  protective reflex, 100
  reflex, afferent pathway, 100
  sequelae, 16
  strength, 158
  testing, 100–101
coughing, 15, 30
crackles
  impact, 15
  right lower lobe, 17
cranial nerve assessment (CNA), 22, 37–39, 44–45
  CSE element, 31
  oromotor assessment (oral exam), 38
  results, **29**
  simplified CNA, **44**
  usage, 39
cranial nerves, 37–39, 44–45, 106, 108
  assessment, **40–43**
  controls, 38
  impact, 12
  involvement, **107**
  origin, 38
  swallowing process, **39**
crepitations
  hearing, 15
  hearing, absence, 25
  right lower lobe, 17
cricoid cartilage (ring-shaped cartilage), 96
cricopharyngeal sphincter
  bolus, contact, 14
  opening, increase, 99–100
  relaxation/opening, suspicion, 60
  upper oesophageal sphincter, 97
cricopharyngeal (upper oesophageal) sphincter, opening, 21
cricopharyngeus, 94
cricothyroid muscles, external laryngeal nerve supply, 96–97
CT scan, usage, 25
cuffed tracheostomy, consideration, 133
cuffless tracheostomy tube in situ, usage, 136
culture, definition, 73–74

D

death, possibility, 148
decannulation, 133–134
  process, **133–134**
decision-making capabilities, 75–76
deep inspiration, 100
dehydration, risks/complications, 148
dementia, **3**
  oral preparatory stage, 13
dentition, 46–47
dentures, problems, 46
depression, occurrence, 70
developmental conditions, 70
diagastric muscles, 96

diagnostic radiographers, 89–90
diaphragmatic breathing, 158
diarrhoea (occurrence), barium ingestion (impact), 144
dietitian
  report, 83
  role, 85
digestive tract, pharynx (sharing), 10–11
direct intervention techniques, **48–51**
direct therapy
  programme, 44
  techniques, 47, 77
disability narrative, 76
discomfort, 94
distress, visibility, 15
drawing skills, honing, 8
drinking
  assistance, 35–36
  barriers, safety, 87
  enabling, 36–37
  enjoyment, loss, 30
  optimal positioning, 112
  risk, 125
drooling, term (usage), 154
drug history (DH), 25, 27
dry mouth (xerostomia), 19, 151–153
dysphagia, 47, 52–53, 66
  acquired dysphagia, 69
  cause, 1
  dehydration, risk, 148
  emphasis, 68–69
  evolution, 92–93
  functional dysphagia, 89
  language, 124
  master's level dysphagia-specific modules, 93
  neurogenic oropharyngeal dysphagia, 161
  possibility, 15
  pre-existing dysphagia, absence, 104
  severity, 70
  temporary dysphagia, 130
  training programme, 86
dysphagia symptoms, 47
  experience, 2
  SOL, impact, 7

E

ear, nose, and throat (ENT), 86
eating
  assistance, 35–36
  enablement, 36–37
  enjoyment, loss, 30, 70
  optimal positioning, 112
  risk, 125
  safety, barriers, 87
eating, confidence
  absence, 64
  improvement, 80
  visual analogue scale, 65
eating, drinking and swallowing (EDS)
  baselines/targets, example, **64**
  client needs, aetiology (understanding), 1
  clinical EDS assessment, 101
  clinician, medical notes (information), **23–24**
  cranial nerves, involvement, **107**
  difficulties, effects, 84
  direct therapy, aim, 47
  EDS-related tasks, 90
  functional EDS symptoms, 7–8
  function, changes (acceptance), 77
  goals, 64, 80
  holistic EDS practice, 68–78
  impairment-based EDS intervention, 66
  intervention, 80
  issues, **3–4**
  practice, 63
  process, cranial nerves (involvement), 38

process, muscles (involvement), 11–12
publications, team investment, 93
quest-driven EDS intervention, 77–78
reflection template, **93**
session plan, **127**
symptoms, absence, 171
symptoms/cause/management strategies, **172**
eating, drinking and swallowing (EDS) assessment, 89, 134–136, 156
risk aversion, 125
telehealth, usage, 157–159
eating, drinking and swallowing (EDS) management, 89, 156
risk aversion, 125
telehealth, usage, 157–159
tenets, 68, 129–130
eating, drinking and swallowing (EDS) needs, 63, 110
addressing, 83
drugs, usage, 88
management, defining, 30
narratives, usage, 75–76
efferent pathways (motor pathways), importance, 105
effortful swallow, 34
Eid-al-Fitr, 72–73
electrical stimulation, 68
electrolytes, dietitian monitoring, 85–86
emotional pain, 76
empathy, tenets, 121
empowering phrase, usage, 75
end of life, 54
comfort/dignity, maintenance, 54
end-of-life care, 54–55
enteral feeding, 55–57, 85
avoidance, 173
choice, MDT decision, 55
client preparation, 2
introduction methods, 5
types, 55–56
usage, 56–57
withdrawal, 57
environment, changes, 35
epiglottic retroversion, 57–58, 115, 147
occurrence, observation, 60
epiglottis, 57–58, 96, 103
base, 123
functioning, compromise, 58
hyoid bone, connection, 57
role, 58
thyroid cartilage, connection, 58
epistaxis, FEES (impact), 62
ethnicity, 74
E-Tran frame, 27
eye-watering, 15

F

false vocal folds, 14
approximation, 95
family social event, 66
fear, occurrence, 70
fenestration, 131
fibreoptic endoscopic evaluation of swallowing (FEES), 16, 32, 60–62
assessment, 21–22
client understanding/ toleration, 62
execution, SLT control, 61
impact, 61
instrumental assessment, 62, 123
objective assessment, 141
portable FEES, usefulness, 61
referral, 164
usage, 58, 60, 147
usage, decision, 61
fibrosis
cause, radiotherapy (impact), 5
stiffening, 58

filtering, 131
fistula (hole), creation, 6
flange, pilot balloon (attachment), 132
fluids
　aspiration, 54–55
　boluses, thickening, 19
　intake, 153
　intake, reduction, 148
　modification, 37
　texture modification, 80
fluoxetine, usage, 164
food
　kosher requirements, 73
　mastication, chewing, 18
　residue, possibility (minimisation), 149
　texture modification, 80
foodstuffs
　availability, 31
　contrast material, mixing, 91
　prohibition, **73**
forced expiration post-swallow, 124
formal training sessions, 35–36
frailty, 148
Frazier Free Water Protocol (Free Water Protocol), 148–149
functional dysphagia, 89
functional EDS symptoms, 7–8
Functional Oral Intake Scale (FOIS), 66
　levels, **66**
functioning, assessment, 67

G

gag reflex, elicitation, 138
gastric pull-up, 7
gastrointestinal tract, focus, 140
general practitioner (GP)
　client referral, 86
　liaison, 37
genioglossus muscle, contraction, 58
Glasgow Coma Scale (GCS), 26

globus, symptom, 8
gloves, usage, 39
goals, **67**
　achievement, intervention (examples), **65**
　baseline/target, 64
　long-term goals/short-term goals, 126
goal-setting, 63–67, 75, 79
gradual-onset dysphagia, trajectory, 2

H

habitual laryngeal penetration, 100
haemoglobin, infrared light absorption, 116
halitosis, 94. 109
head and neck
　cancer, radiotherapy (usage), 56, 152
　SOL treatment, 2, 5
head/body positioning, 32–33
　advantages/disadvantages, 33
head/body positions, rationale (inclusion), **33**
head injury, 35
　severity, 656
head positions, 69, 124
　alteration, impact, 32–33
　changes, 113
　client understanding, 36
　compensatory strategies, 7
　strategies, 123
　testing, 61
headrests, usage, 113
Health and Care Professions Council (HCPC), *One Chance to Get it Right*, 54
healthcare
　assistant, role, 86
　depersonalisation, 68
health status, changes, 86–87
heart valves, inflammation, 110

heat and moisture exchange (HME) device, usage, 131
hemiparesis (body weakness), 112
  presence, 161
hemiplegia (body paralysis), 112
hiatus hernia, presence, 25
high temperature (pyrexia), 17
Hillsborough disaster, anoxic brain injury (sustaining), 57
History of presenting condition (HPC), 25, 26
holism, 74–75
holistic EDS practice, 68–78
  chaos, 76
  cultural aspects, 73–74
  power differential, mitigation, 74–75
  psychological aspects, 69–70
  quest, 77–78
  restitution, 76–77
  social aspects, 71
  spiritual/religious aspects, 71–73
holistic practice, 75
Holy Communion (Eucharist), taking, 72, 85
humidification, 131
Huntington's disease, 2, **4**
hydration
  dietitian monitoring, 85–86
  human need, 57
hyoepiglottic ligament, 57
hyoglossus muscles, usage, 96
hyoid bone
  larynx boundary, 96
  middle finger, usage, 98
  thyroid cartilage, connection, 58
hyolaryngeal excursion, 14, 97
  impairment, 97
  treatment options, 99–100
hyoscine, usage, 154
hypertension
  past medical history, 160–161
  presence, 25

hypopharynx, 10
  bolus, transfer, 21
hypoxaemia (low oxygen levels), indication, 116

I

illness
  narratives, 75, 76
  patient, passive subject, 76–77
  physical aspects, 69
impairment, 79
impairment-based intervention, 68–69
incisors, comprising, 46
infection, signs, 22
  absence, 170
inferior pharyngeal constrictors, 94
information-gathering, 22, 63
  tracheostomy, 135
information, salient pieces (identification), 27
inhaled air, humidification, 131
inner cannula, removal/washing/ replacement, 131
innervation, 151–152
instrumental assessments, 61
instrumental assessment technique, 5
  usage, 32, 134
internal laryngeal nerves, supply, 96–97
International Classification of Disability, Functioning and Health (ICF)
  framework, usage, 63
  health domains, **79**
  influence, 79
International Dysphagia Diet Standardisation Initiative (IDDSI), 80–81, 161
  standards/testing methods, 80
International Dysphagia Diet Standardisation Initiative (IDDSI) levels, 36, 37
  descriptions/examples, **81**

management, 65
recommendations, 19, 164
intervention
　aim, 2
　plan, 31
intra-oral pressure, 13
intra-oral sensation, reduction, 122
intrinsic laryngeal muscles, presence, 96
invasive techniques, usage, 88–89
ionising radiation
　client exposure/inappropriateness, MDT perspective, 61
　overexposure, 90
　risks, 125, 146
Iowa Oral Performance Instrument (IOPI®), 80
IQoro®, 80
ischaemic damage, CT scan (usage), 25
IX cranial nerve (glossopharyngeal nerve), 151, 160
　control, 38

J

joint sessions, usage, 83
Joint working, 83–91
journal articles, reading/summarising, 93
Judaism, food (kosher requirements), 73

K

Killian's dehiscence, 94
Killian's triangle, 94
kyphosis, 98
　presence, 112
　severity, 145

L

language
　challenges, 135
　patient requirement, 141
　power, 68
laryngeal anatomy/physiology/function/innervation, 95–97
laryngeal cancer, larynx removal, 99
laryngeal excursion, 97
laryngeal palpation, 29, 38, 97–99
　CSE element, 31
　execution, 101
　finger placement, **98**
　possibility, absence, 135
laryngeal penetration, 15–17, 60
　episodes, experiencing, 70
　experience, 16
　indications, 173
laryngeal vestibule, 95
　entrance, covering, 58
　entrance, narrowing, 33
　penetration, 16
laryngectomy
　stoma, creation, 130
　tracheostomy, EDS differences, 137
laryngopharynx, 10
laryngospasm, FEES (impact), 62
larynx, 95–101
　cancer, surgical removal (importance), 5
　cartilages, 96
　function, assessment, 95
　innervation, 96–97
　movement, 98
　removal, 6–7, 99
　structures, observation, 61
lateral cricoarytenoid muscles, 96
lateral jaw movement, reduction, 37
late-stage dementia
　enteral feeding, usage, 56–57
　population, ethical issues, 57
laughing, avoidance, 36
lead aprons, wearing, 147

lead gauntlet, usage, 146
learning, 92–93
  deepening, 158
  disability, 8
Lee Silverman Voice Treatment® (LSVT), 51
left parotid salivary gland, radiotherapy (usage), 30
left-sided hemiparesis, 25
lesion, site, 164
Levodopa, usage, 88
lifelong difficulties, experiencing, 69–70
lingual control, 122
lip moistening gels, usage, 111
lip seal
  buccal tension, combination, 152
  reduction, 158
lips, oral mucosa, 151
lisinopril, usage, 164
local choking policies, 16
long-term goals, 126
loss, sense, 70
lower face, muscle (origin), 19
lower-frequency sounds, usage, 21
lower motor neurone signs, evidence, 164
lunchtime assessments, 35

M

mandible
  movement, 13
  necrosis, development (risk), 46
  reconstruction, 5
Masako exercise, 50
mask-like structure, 5
master's level dysphagia-specific modules, 93
mastication (chewing), 13, 103
  difficulty, 18–19
  reduction, 37
maxilla (necrosis), development (risk), 46

mealtimes
  distractibility, 52–53
  talking/laughing, avoidance, 36
medical notes, information, **23–24**
medication, 103–104
  EDS-related side effects, **104**
  positive effects, 104
memory, pain, 68
Mendelsohn manoeuvre, 158
Mental Capacity Act (2005), 146
Microsoft Teams, usage, 83
milk seepage, signs, 6
minor salivary glands, 151
mobility, reduction, 148
modified barium swallow, 140
Modified Barium Swallow Impairment Profile™, 147
Modified Evans Blue Dye Test (MEBDT), 136
molars, usage, 46
motor neurone disease, 2, **4**, 59
mouth-breathing, impact, 152
mouthcare
  importance, 55
  optimum, 54
mouth hydrator, usage, 55
mouth, opening, 13
  reduction, 30
mucin (lubricant-type protein), 151
mucositis
  cause, radiotherapy (impact), 5
  suffering, 46
mucous membrane, inflammation, 138
mucous-type saliva, function, 152
multidisciplinary team (MDT), 156
  decisions, 55
  questions, 120
muscle weakness (sarcopenia), 114

musculoskeletal system, assessment/management, 88

N

nasendoscope, usage, 61
nasogastric tube (NGT), 6
  enteral feeding type, 55
  usage, 70, 170
nasopharynx, 10
neck
  cancer, radiotherapy (usage), 56, 152
  SOL treatment, 2, 5
neurodegenerative conditions, 2, 56
  impact, 103
neurodegenerative diagnosis, 171
neurogenic aetiologies, 1–2
neurogenic conditions, 1–2
neurogenic oropharyngeal dysphagia, 161
  presentation, 170, 173
neurological conditions, EDS issues, **3–4**
neurological impairment, 100
neurological pathology, 114
neurological recovery, 44
neurological system, assessment/management, 88
neurological underpinnings, 12, 105–108
neuromuscular electrical stimulation (NMES), 51
nil by mouth (NBM), 5, 25, 27, 105, 148, 170
nil per os (NPO), 105
non-dominant hemisphere, stroke (occurrence), 160
non-foaming toothpaste, usage, 111
non-insulin-dependent diabetes mellitus (NIDDM), 27
non-invasive techniques, usage, 88
non-maleficence, biomedical ethical principle, 124
non-verbal oral apraxia, 45
nucleus ambiguus, efferent messages, 105–106
nurse, role/responsibility, 86–87
nutrients, derivation, 54–55
nutrition
  derivation, 70
  human need, 57
nutritional intake, artificial method, 55
nutrition/hydration (EDS management tenet), 68, 114, 129

O

observation (CSE element), 31
occupational therapist (OT)
  joint-working, 36–37
  role, 87
occupational therapy, usage, 112
odynophagia, 109, 115
oedema (swelling), subsidence, 5, 160
oesophageal stage, 15, 140
oesophagectomy, 7
oesophagus
  bolus, approach, 14
  bolus, entry, 97
  collapse, 11
  dilation, 11, 15
  direction, 95
  muscular contraction (peristalsis), 11
older clients, dentures, 46
One Chance to Get it Right (HCPC), 54
one-way valve, 131
on examination (O/E), 27
oral bacteria
  impact, 148
  presence, 109
oral care, 109–111
  nursing duty, 111

oral cavity
  bolus path, 140
  bolus/saliva, presence, 19
  decay, 46
  food/fluid entry, 13
  food residue, possibility (minimisation), 149
oral examination, 109–111
oral hygiene, 31, 109–111
  concerns, **110**
  exam, results, 28
  problem, 110
Oralieve®, 55
oral intake, 69–70
oral intake, aspiration, 59
  likelihood, assessment, 31
oral musculature, tension, 13
oral preparatory stage, 12–13, 140, 161
  assessment, 143
  bypassing, 35
  direct intervention techniques, **48–49**
  food, mastication, 18
  oral stage, combination, 12
  prolongation, 29
  usage, 12–13
oral residue, 122–123
  absence, 29, 30
  assessment, 122–123
oral stage, 13–14, 144, 161
  assessment, 143
  oral preparatory stage, combination, 12
oral thrush, 109
oral transit time (OTT), 14
oral trials, 38, 113
  avoidance, 44
  commencement, prohibitions, 73
  CSE element, 31
  rationale, **32**
  result, 29–31
  usage, 15
orofacial musculature, 158
orofacial symmetry, 31

oromotor assessment (oral exam), 38, 158
oromotor exercises, 90
  implementation, 171
oropharynx, 10
osteophytes, 114–116
  complaints, 115
  idiopathic characteristics, 115
  pain management, 109
  presence, 115
osteoradionecrosis, 46
outcomes, **67**
  measurement, 63–67, 79
outer cannula, 131
overt aspiration, visualisation, 62
oxygen saturation, 116
  reduction, 170

P

palpation, usage, 98
Panther, Kathy, 148
parenteral feeding, 85
  reference, 56
Parkinson's disease, 2, **4**
  EDS needs, client mapping, **79**
  Levodopa, usage, 88
  pharyngeal stage, relationship, 14
parotid glands, location, 151
Passavant's ridge, 14
  meeting, 138
  pad, 14
passivity, language (usage), 76–77
past medical history (PMH), 25, 27
  results, 164
pathology, absence, 7–8
Penetration/Aspiration Scale, 141
  basis, **142–143**
pen torch, usage, 39
percutaneous endoscopic gastrostomy (PEG), 70, 109, 173
  enteral feeding type, 56

percutaneous endoscopic jejunostomy (PEJ), enteral feeding type, 56
periodontal disease, association, 110
peripheral nervous system, formation, 37–38
peristalsis, 11
personalised care, promotion, 68
person-centred goals, 31
promotion, 68
Phagenyx®, 51
pharmacist, role, 87–88
pharyngeal contraction, reduction, 114
pharyngeal pouch (Zenker's diverticulum), 94
pharyngeal residue, 123–124
management strategies, 123–124
post-swallow, 123
pharyngeal stage, 14, 161
difficulties (targeting), direct intervention techniques (usage), **50–51**
issues, gauging (difficulty), 143
pharyngeal structures, observation, 60
pharyngeal transit time (PTT), 14
pharyngeal wall, contact, 138
pharynx, 131
constriction, 39
direction, 95
division, 10–11
food/fluid, pooling, 21
food residue, possibility (minimisation), 149
pooling/residue, suspicion, 60
structures, observation, 61
physical disability, 8
physical health, maintenance, 72
physical need, 129
physical pain, 76
physiology, 8–15
alteration, 115
musculature, 11–12
oesophageal stage, 15
oral preparatory stage, 12–13
oral stage, 13–14
pharyngeal stage, 14
structures, 9–11
physiotherapist, role, 88
physiotherapist (respiratory), role, 88–89
physiotherapy, usage, 112
piecemeal deglutition, 4, 18
pillows, usage, 113
polypharmacy, 148
positioning, 98, 112–114
posterior cricoarytenoid muscles, abduction, 96
posterior tracheal wall, anterior oesophageal wall (fistula creation), 6
post-swallow glottal release, 21
posture, observation, 158
power differential, mitigation, 74–75
power, wielding, 75–76
pre-existing dysphagia, absence, 104
pre-existing pathologies, evidence (absence), 161
premolars, usage, 46
presbyphagia, 8, 114–116
presenting condition (PC), 160–161
productive cough, 17
profiling beds, usage, 113
prognosis, need, 77
progressive disorders, 59
protective cough, initiation, 96–97
psychological burden, 70
psychological therapy, usage, 8
psychologist, role, 89
pulmonary function, reduction, 116

pulse oximetry, 16, 116
  usage, 60
pure water, usage, 150
pyrexia (high temperature), 17
pyriform fossae (pear-shaped fossae), 123
pyriform sinuses, observation, 61

Q

quality of life (EDS management tenet), 68, 114, 129
quest-driven EDS intervention, 77–78
questions, **118–119**, 118–120

R

radiographer, role, 89–90
radiologically inserted gastrostomy, enteral feeding type, 56
radiologist, role, 89
radio-opaque contrast material, usage, 141
radiotherapy
  effects, subsiding, 109
  usage, 5, 30, 46, 56
radiotherapy-induced mucositis, 109
Ramadan, fasting, 72–73
recovery, hope (absence), 76
recurrent laryngeal nerve (CN X)
  branching, 97
  damage, 7
  ipsilateral branch, 97
reflection, 92–93
  frameworks, usage, 92
  template (EDS), **93**
reflux, client complaint, 6
regurgitation, 94
rehabilitation, 56
religious groups, prohibited foodstuffs, **73**
religious rites, impact, 84–85
residual orofacial weakness, display, 38
residual weakness, 38
residue, 122–124
  accumulation, 114
  creation, 97
  visuo-perceptual judgements, 143
residue/pooling, 60
respiration, ventilator support, 132
respiratory physiotherapist, role, 88–89
respiratory tract, pharynx (sharing), 10–11
restitution, 76–77
  narrative, 77
right frontotemporal area, ischaemic damage (evidence), 25
right hemisphere stroke, 25
right lower lobe, crackles/crepitations, 17
right-sided hemianopia, 35
risk, 124–125
role, sense (impacts), 70

S

sarcopenia (age-related muscle weakness), 114
safety (EDS management tenet), 68, 114, 129
salbutamol, usage, 164
saliva
  anterior escape, evidence, 158
  control, 31
  excess (sialorrhoea), 151, 153–154
  function, 152
  production, impacts, 152
  production, reduction/increase, **88**
  reduction, 30, 46
  viscosity, changes, 19
salivation, 151
sarcopenic individuals, presence, 101
seating posture, 75
secretions, management, 54

self, sense (impacts), 70
sensory information, impact, 12
sensory nerve fibres, 100
sensory neurones, 106
sepsis, 148
session plan
  components, 126
  EDS, **127**
session planning, 126
Shaker exercise, aim, 99–100
short-term goals, 126
sialorrhoea, 19, 151, 153–154
signage, creation, 90
silent aspiration, 17
  diagnosis, VF/FEES usage, 143
  suspicion, 141
skin, breakdown, 130
smoking, history, 148
smooth muscle contractions (peristalsis), 15
social events, 71
social history (SH), 27
socialisation, 70
soft toothbrushes, usage, 111
solid consistency, trialling, 141
soreness, 109
space-occupying lesion (SOL), 2
  impact, 7
specific, measurable, appropriate/achievable, realistic/relevant, and timebound (SMART), 63–65
speech and language therapist (SLT)
  assessment toolkit, 21
  clients, enteral feeding (usage), 56
  community work, 83
  CSE, usage, 31
  decision, absence, 105
  diagnosis, 22
  diagnostic categories, 66
  dietitian, liaison, 85
  end-of-life care, 55
  guidance, 91
  intervention-planning, ICF influence, 79
  liaison, 6
  monitoring, requirement, 5
  oral trials assessment, 155
  outpatient clinic, client attendance, 86
  patient interaction, 98
  practice, spirituality (consideration), 71
  questions, **28**
  recommendations, checking, 36
  role, 54–55, 57, 59
  service, 37
  video, provision, 35
speech and language therapy
  assistant, role, 90
  student, role, 90–91
speech, changes, 30
spine, curvature, 112
spirituality, consideration, 71
spiritual pain, 76
spiritual resources, client access, 71
spontaneous swallows
  number, reduction, 153
  observation, 31
stakeholders, intervention outcome (display), 66
starch-based thickening agent, usage, 151
step-up/step-down activities, 126
sternohyoid muscles, 96
sternothyroid muscles, 96
stethoscope
  bell/diaphragm, cleaning, 21
  usage, 21
stimulation techniques, 90
stomach ulcers, diagnosis, 140
stoma, creation, 130
stripping motion, 13
stroke
  occurrence, 160
structural dysphagia, occurrence, 2, 5

structural pathology, 114
stylohyoid muscles, 96
subglottic pressure, normalisation, 131
subjectivity, propensity, 80
submental tissue, excess, 98
sudden-onset EDS issues, 1–2
sulci, sweep, 123
super-supraglottic swallow, 124
supplementation, adjustments, 85
support/supervision, 155–156
suppository, usage, 103
supraglottic region, 95
supraglottic swallow, 100, 124
suprahyoid muscles
  links, 96
  strengthening, 99–100
surface electromyography (sEMG), 51
swallow
  anatomy, tracheostomy tube (impact), 135
  clinical assessment, 108
  difficulties, possibility, **52**
  effort, 124
  elicitation, 30
  exercise, 100
  function, explanation, 144
  larynx, movement, 98
  observation, 19, 36
  oral preparatory phases, 19, 46
  stages, 47
  trigger, delay, 33, 60
  volitional stages, 106
swallowing
  assessment/management, 161
  effort/pain, 30
  initiation, oral preparatory stage (usage), 12–13
  oral preparatory stage, 103, 138
  pain, 116
  position, 99–100, 113
  recommendations, 112
swallowing, musculature
  innervation, cranial nerves (impact), 12
  involvement, **11–12**
swallowing process, 58
  breakdown, 149
  cranial nerves, involvement, **39**
swallowing strategies, 124
  safety, 87
  testing, 61
swallow manoeuvres, 34–35, 158
  rationale, inclusion, **34**
swallow physiology
  alteration, 68–69
  changes, 173
  improvement, 47
  therapeutic effects, 18–19
  tracheostomy tube, impact, 135
swallow process
  anatomical structures, **9–10**
  anatomy/physiology, visualisation (objective method), 140
  medications, impact, 104
  tracheostomy presence, impact, **132**
swallow reflex, 58, 61, 103, 114
  delay, 30
  stimulation, 68
  triggering, 39
Swedish nose, 131
symptomatic therapy, usage, 8

T

talking, avoidance, 36
tastes for pleasure, 129
tele-assessment/tele-management, selection (reasons), 157
telehealth, usage, 157–159
telephone, usage, 83
temperature stimulation, 68
temporary dysphagia, 130
texture modification, 33, 37

therapeutic head/body positions, **113**
therapeutic radiographers, 89–90
therapy goals, 66
Therapy Outcome Measures (TOMs), 66, 67
  basis, 80
throat
  stethoscope, usage, 21
thyroepiglottic ligament, 58
thyrohyoid ligament, 58
thyrohyoid muscles, 96
thyrohyoid shortening, enhancement, 100
thyroid cartilage (shield-shaped cartilage), 96
  little finger, usage, 98
  ring finger, usage, 98
thyroid shield, usage, 146, 147
Timed Water Swallow Test (TWST), 149
tissue, fibrosis, 5
tongue
  base, observation, 61
  blue dye, placement, 136
  depressor, usage, 39
tongue movement
  reduction, 122
  slowness, 30
tongue-pumping, 29
toothbrushing (NHS recommendation), 47
tooth extraction, requirement, 46
trachea, 130
  food/fluid/saliva, entry, 15
  observation, 61
  oesophagus, separation, 5–6
tracheostomised client
  assessment, 134
  MEBDT, usage, 136
tracheostomy, 91, 130–137
  case history-taking, problems, 135
  cuffless tracheostomy tube in situ, usage, 136
  cuff, usage, 132
  EDS assessment, 134–136
  EDS difficulties, fistula creation (relationship), 137
  EDS management, 136
  information-gathering, 135
  laryngectomy, EDS differences, 137
  voicing, impossibility, 130–131
tracheostomy tube
  cuffed, 132
  insertion, 2, 5, 130
  presence, impact, **132**
  presence, issues (mitigation), **135**
  removal, 134
transient ischaemic attack (TIA), history, 25
traumatic brain injury, **3**
treatment centres, usage, 115
trismus (cause), radiotherapy (impact), 5
true vocal folds, closure, 95
trust, essence, 118
two-pronged clinical approach, 8

U

unconditional positive regard, tenets, 121
unilateral innervation, 106
unilateral pooling/residue, 123
unilateral stroke, **3**
unilateral upper motor neurone dysarthria, 160
upper motor neurones (UMNs), 106, 108
  evidence, 164
upper oesophageal sphincter (cricopharyngeal sphincter), bolus (contact), 14
urinary tract infections, 148
utensils, 36–37

uvula, 138
uvulitis, occurrence, 138

V

vagus nerve, 97
  sensory nerve fibres, 100
valleculae
  closure, 33
  formation, 58
  post-swallow, 123
  residue, accumulation, 114
vallecular residue, post-swallow evidence, 143
valve, failure, 6
V cranial nerve (trigeminal nerve), 160
  control, 38, 106
velopharyngeal closure, compromise, 138
velopharyngeal incompetence, suspicion, 61
velum (soft palate), rise, 14
vestibular folds, 95
victimhood, language (usage), 76
videofluoroscopy (VF), 140–147
  assessment, 21–22
  biofeedback tool, 33
  C-arm, positioning, 140–141
  clinic, 89–90
  clinic, SLT control, 145
  consent, 145–146
  head positions, trialling, 144
  instrumental assessment, 123
  ionising radiation, precautions/risks, 146
  measurements, **142**
  objective assessment, 141
  personnel, roles, **145**
  preclusion, pregnancy (relationship), 147
  procedure, 140–143
  procedure, preclusion, 144–145
  pros/cons, 144–145
  real-time moving images, usage, 140
  referral, 164
  report, writing, 147
  results, 125
  safety considerations, 146–147
  side effects, possibility (avoidance), 61
  usage, 5, 14, 58, 60, 91, 115
  usage, suggestion, 171
  usefulness, 35
VII cranial nerve (facial nerve), 152
  control, 38, 106
visual analogue scale, 65
vocal folds. *See also* false vocal folds
  abduction, 95
  abduction, posterior cricoarytenoid muscles (impact), 96
  adduction, 14
  length, alteration, 97
  length/tension/thickness, 96
  level, 130
  observation, 61
  protection, 96
  true vocal folds, closure, 95
vocalising ability, 27
vocal quality, 31, 158
voice
  ability, facilitation, 131
  restoration valve, 99
voicing, impossibility, 130–131

W

water
  Frazier Free Water Protocol (Free Water Protocol), 148–149
  protocols/tests, 148–150
  pure water, usage, 150
  Timed Water Swallow Test (TWST), 149
weight loss, 30, 83
wet voice, 15
wheelchair trays, usage, 113

white cell count (WCC)
    absence, 2, 275
    increase, 17
white-out, occurrence, 62

X

X cranial nerve (vagal nerve), 160
    control, 38, 106, 138
xerostomia (dry mouth), 19, 151–153
    after-effects, 153
    cause, 164
    cause, radiotherapy (impact), 5
XI cranial nerve (accessory nerve), 107
XII cranial nerve (hypoglossal nerve), control, 38, 106

X-ray, 115
    chest X-rays, interpretation/reading, 88, 89
    guidance, 56
    real-time moving images, usage, 140
    source/detector, usage, 141
    suite, client perception, 147
    usage, 5

Y

yoghurt, usage, 29, 31, 155
your support/supervision, 155–156

Z

Zenker's diverticulum, 94
Zoom
    usage, 157–159

For Product Safety Concerns and Information please contact our EU
representative GPSR@taylorandfrancis.com
Taylor & Francis Verlag GmbH, Kaufingerstraße 24, 80331 München, Germany

www.ingramcontent.com/pod-product-compliance
Lightning Source LLC
Chambersburg PA
CBHW060605230426
43670CB00011B/1980